W9-ABM-955

RUN FOR GOD®

DEVOTIONS

Finding God in a Runners Space

Volume Two

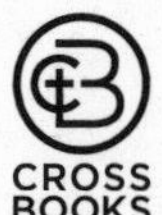

VISIT RUN FOR GOD ONLINE AT www.RunforGod.com

ISBN: 9781462744824 (Hard Cover)

ISBN: 9781462744831 (Soft Cover)

Library of Congress Control Number: 2014916619

Printed in the United States of America by Crossbooks Publishing, a division of Lifeway.

If you require medical, fitness, or nutritional advice, you must contact your own health care professional. You should seek the advice of a doctor before starting any exercise routine.

This book may contain information relating to various medical conditions and their treatment and an exercise/nutrition protocol. Such information is provided for informational purposes only and is not meant to be a substitute for the advice of a physician or health care professional. You should not use this information for diagnosing or treating a health problem or injury.

To make informed health care decisions, you should always consult your physician for your personal medical needs. Neither Run for God nor its agents, affiliates, partners, or licensors are providing these materials to you for the purpose of giving you medical advice.

For any questions about your health and well-being, please consult your physician.

Table of Contents

before you get started

The Thing about a Shirt

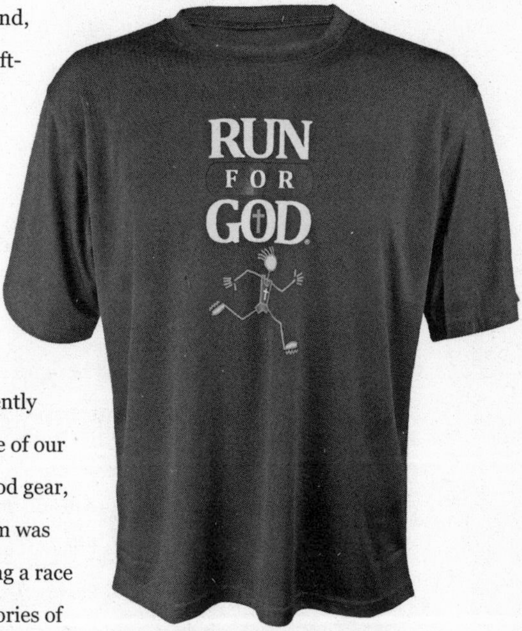

A FEW YEARS BACK I WAS in Richmond, Virginia, for the Youth and Junior Elite Ddraft-Legal Triathlon. Some of our young athletes were competing, and it was an all-around great trip. Something happened this weekend that happens quite often to our entire Run for God family. A gentleman went out of his way to comment on our shirts, specifically, the kids' Run for God Triathlon Suits. He said that his son had recently come to know the Lord, and when he saw one of our athletes on the course wearing his Run for God gear, it inspired him. The other part of our Tri team was competing at another venue, and while getting a race summary from that venue, I heard similar stories of people commenting on the Run for God tent and shirts. On the eight-hour drive home, I pulled up my Facebook and began reading how Ben Reed, an instructor in Westerville, Ohio, had volunteered his class to work the packet pick-up at a local race where 14,500 runners were present. Guess what? They were all wearing their Run for God shirts, and to hear the impact they had on those runners was awesome.

I wear a Run for God shirt 95% of the time, and I get many comments from many people. The vast majority of comments are great, inspiring, and the type that let me know that the Lord has reached down and touched someone's day, even if it's just a small touch. Others are witty and sometimes rude, like the guy who asked me "What's God running for—President?" I'm convinced that even those people are touched in some way.

Can a t-shirt make a difference? I say yes, but I say that with a strong word of caution. People today seem to be more aware than ever of how others handle and portray themselves. A Run for God shirt, or any spiritual shirt for that matter, on the shoulders of someone who is out in the world living for Christ and reflecting Jesus can be a very powerful thing. It says a lot about who you are and whom you follow. It lets others know what you stand for without you ever having to open your mouth. But you must be walking with Christ and reflecting His light for that shirt to have any power.

I have a friend that had a quote printed on the back of his Run for God shirt: "Preach the Gospel, and if necessary, use words." That statement is so true! We can talk all we want about how we live for God and even have a closet full of spiritual shirts, but if our actions do not back up what we are representing, then we are only hurting the cause and our words have no validity.

"Now then, we are ambassadors for Christ, as though God were pleading through us: we implore you on Christ's behalf, be reconciled to God. For He made Him who knew no sin to be sin for us, that we might become the righteousness of God in Him" (2 Corinthians 5:20–21).

Get your shirt at **www.RunforGod.com**

"Preach the Gospel, and if necessary, use words."

getting started

WE HOPE YOU'LL ENJOY READING RUN for God—Devotions as much as we enjoyed putting it together. Devotions came together as a result of the outpouring of letters and e-mails that come into the Run for God camp each week. These stories of ordinary people doing extraordinary things and Run for God's role in their lives prompted us to find a way to preserve these memories. From a desire to both preserve and share these stories, Devotions was born.

This Bible study is not your ordinary study. No, it's a study that is made up of stories from people just like you and me, real stories from real people. These thoughts and experiences are brought to you from pastors, deacons, Sunday school teachers, new Christians, old Christians, and even Christians who had lost their way for a time. So if you're looking for a study that is authored by a renowned theologian, this isn't it. But if you're looking for a study that shows what God can do through someone just like you or me, then you've definitely come to the right place.

So how do you use this book? I'm glad you asked. Devotions is designed to be a weekly one-year study in which you tackle a task each weekday and recap on the weekends. Let me just lay out a typical week for you.

Monday *Read the main story.*
Tuesday *Look up and study the scriptures provided.*
Wednesday *Write down, recite, and commit to memory the verses of the week.*
Thursday *Ponder and write down your response to the questions of the week.*
Friday *Read "Running Observations by Dean." You're going to love this guy!*

Weekend *Recap and journal your thoughts from the previous week in your Sticky Notes.*

You may be wondering if this study could be used in small groups? You bet! While we have **5K**, **10K**, and **Half Marathon Challenges** that are designed for small group settings, you may be part of a running club full of seasoned runners or a Run for God class that has graduated from all the Challenges. Whichever the case may be, grab some friends, agree on a time to get together each week, share the study, and hold each other accountable for your training. Feel free to use the training schedules located in the back of the book as a workout guide.

I think you now have all the tools to get started. From all of us here at **Run for God**, we hope you enjoy this study. Should you need anything, or if you have a story you'd like to share, feel free to reach out to us at **www.RunforGod.com**.

Keep pointing people to Jesus!
Mitchell Hollis

who is dean?

DEAN THOMPSON IS A GREAT FRIEND of the Run for God ministry and a really fast runner. While we were planning this Devotions project, we wanted the input of someone who was both a veteran to the sport of running and very open about his relationship with Christ. It didn't take very long to decide he was the man for the job.

Our challenge to Dean was very simple. Take the most common topics that you discuss with runners and non-runners alike, and tell us about them in your own words. I think that you will find Dean's thoughts inspiring, informational, and even funny at times. Needless to say, we think Dean is a pretty cool guy.

Here's a little more about Dean as told by his wife Debbie.

"Running is the only thing I'm good at." I've heard Dean say these words many times, but they simply are not true.

Born in Perth Amboy, New Jersey, Dean's family moved to Miami, Florida, when he was five years old. This is where his running career began.

He and his family lived in one of the large mobile home parks in Miami. In fact, the park was so large that the Thompson's home sat on Lot # Z15. When Dean's mother drove to the park's post office to pick up their mail, Dean wouldn't ride in the car. He would run in front of the car all the way to the post office and back home again. With every trip to the post office, Dean's competitiveness would kick in, pushing him to run faster than he did in his last "race against mom's car."

He played baseball while attending Flamingo Elementary and Redland Elementary schools in Florida and continued to play after his family moved to Riverdale, Georgia, when he was 10 years old. He always led his team in stolen bases. "I was offended if anyone got close to my total," he said. "When someone got close, I'd just steal more bases." He was a true runner, even on the baseball field.

While in the ninth grade, he tried out for the track team, running a 5:31 mile in his first-ever timed mile and securing a place on the team. He ran the 880, the mile, and the mile relay, finishing second in the county for the mile, losing by one-hundredth of a second. In his sophomore year, he began running with the cross-country team. Leading his first JV 5K race, a volunteer pointed him in the wrong direction. He soon recognized this, turned around, and still finished in second place. He continued to run through his junior and senior years and was named to the 2nd All-Southeastern Cross Country Team. He won a state championship in cross-country and two state championships in track. After high school, he attended Georgia Tech on an athletic scholarship, running both cross-country and track.

Dean continued to run after college, but it wasn't until he turned forty that he began to get serious again. He has run the Boston Marathon two times and the Myrtle Beach Marathon three times, winning the race in 2013. He runs numerous local races in the North Georgia and Chattanooga areas. He is also a member of the Chattanooga Track Club Masters team that competes nationally.

While his passion for running is obvious, so is his love for our Lord. I see this passion as he encourages other runners, including myself, to do their best in a race. He is always eager to talk with people about running as well as their walk with Christ. Recognizing that our love for each other is strengthened by our love for our Lord, we are very active in our church and community.

So when Dean says that running is the only thing at which he's good, I have to politely disagree. He is also a good husband, father, athlete, and encourager, giving God the glory while pressing on toward the goal for the prize of the upward call of God in Christ Jesus (Philippians 3:14).

inactivity and fear lead to a dangerous path

THE JOURNEY TO MY NEW LIFE began in April of 2013. At that time, I was weighing in at over 300 pounds and climbing fast. I had no energy to become a healthier person. I had no energy to even play with my children. I tried to never outwardly let my family or friends see the disappointment that I was feeling on the inside. How did I let myself get to this point? Why did I never ask for help? What can I do to change? God heard my questions and silent cries for help. He began answering them long before I realized that I was asking them.

In the fall of 2012, my wife signed up to take the Run for God 5K Challenge in Cape Girardeau, Missouri. Already an active and fit person, I really paid no attention to her becoming a runner. I always support her, but this wasn't something that I had any interest in personally. As the weeks passed, I watched her become a stronger runner, but noticed a bigger change in her. She was becoming a better Christian. She was talking to people more about running and faith. She was telling anyone who would listen, and sometimes those who wouldn't (me), about the similarities between enduring a race, and having an enduring faith. After she crossed the finish line at the graduation race, the joy on her face was indescribable, but the growing joy in her heart was overwhelming. I began to wonder why I was being so hesitant to join her, even though I knew the answer, fear. I was afraid it was going to hurt. I was afraid I would look foolish. I was afraid of failure.

When she told me she felt led to lead her own group in the spring, I couldn't have been happier for her. I knew how important this was to her. Then she asked me to join her. I immediately resisted. Fear had a firm grip on me, with no intentions of letting go. She asked me to pray about it, which admittedly, I didn't do nearly enough. After several weeks of serious thought and prayer, and asking myself those questions above, I agreed to try. I felt that this was the answer for which I was secretly looking. God was revealing His plan to me, and all I had to do was follow Him.

On the first day of Run for God in Anna-Jonesboro, Illinois, I was amazed to see so many people like myself. Everyone there had his or her own story. Everyone had his or her own struggles, and reasons for being there. It was reassuring to me to see I wasn't alone. I was immediately glad that I chose to listen and trust in the Lord. One by one, my fears were put to rest. I found out quickly that it did hurt. There was no way around that. I was very heavy, and was doing something with my body that I hadn't done in a very long time. As far as looking foolish, I guess that's in the eye of the beholder. I'm sure it was a sight seeing a 300 pound man trudging away step after step, and while some may have viewed that as comical or foolish, my hope was that others might be able to draw inspiration from it, or in the very least, ask me why I was doing it, so I could tell them all about Run for God and what it was doing for me and my family. Once I made the commitment to join the challenge, failure was no longer an option. How could I fail with God, and so many amazing people running alongside me? How can anyone be a failure when he has faith?

Week after week, I found myself talking to God more and talking to people about Him a lot more. I was excited to tell people how my health and my faith were improving because of Run for God. I began looking for chances to witness to people, when before, someone might not have even been able to tell that I was a Christian. After I crossed the finish line at my graduation race, I knew the same joy that my wife had felt just a few months before. I could see that joy in myself now. I was no longer feeling the shame and disappointment that I had felt just weeks before. I had a new confidence in myself, and a renewed commitment to Jesus. Since that day, I've run in six 5k's, two 10 milers, two half marathons, and a full marathon. None of this would have been possible for me had it not been for Run for God, and some really special people. Thank you.

David Whitaker – *Jonesboro, IL*

get in the word

Isaiah 40:31
But those who wait on the Lord shall renew their strength; they shall mount up with wings like eagles, they shall run and not be weary, they shall walk and not faint.

Hebrews 12:1-3
Therefore we also, since we are surrounded by so great a cloud of witnesses, let us lay aside every weight, and the sin which so easily ensnares us, and let us run with endurance the race that is set before us, looking unto Jesus, the author and finisher of our faith, who for the joy that was set before Him endured the cross, despising the shame, and has sat down at the right hand of the throne of God. For consider Him who endured such hostility from sinners against Himself, lest you become weary and discouraged in your souls.

Romans 5:3-4

And not only that, but we also glory in tribulations, knowing that tribulation produces perseverance; and perseverance, character; and character, hope.

TRibulations
Perseverancy
Charactor
hope

scripture memorization

Write out the scripture(s) in the space below and recite them ten times.

ESIAH 40:31 But Those who wait upon The Lord shall Renew
them strength; They shall mount up with wings like Eagles
ey shall Run and not be weary They shall walk and
ot faint.

TRibulations - Produces persenverance,
Character, hope

something to ponder

HOW CAN this challenge make me a better disciple?

WILL I continue this lifestyle after the Run for God class is complete?

WHAT IS my main goal throughout this entire process?

running observations by Dean

I Can't Do That

I WAS RECENTLY AT A FRIEND'S house when, in the course of our discussion, he thought about a video that he had seen of high school kids doing amazing exercises. We went to his computer, queued the video and watched as these students from the 1950s performed exercises on parallel bars and on the ground that were very impressive. Perhaps the most astonishing thing about the video was the number of students who were in such great shape and could perform these tough exercises. One procedure that looked particularly difficult and did not require any equipment to perform caught our eye. I would find out later that it is known as a Lalanne Pushup, named for the famous fitness expert of that era. It is basically a pushup with your arms stretched out in front of you like superman.

There were teenagers and younger kids at the house who decided they would try to perform these pushups. I watched as these kids, who are good athletes, laid on the floor with arms outstretched and tried to push their bodies up off the floor. No one moved. Then I watched as an adult tried it and couldn't do it, and this was a good swimmer who, in all likelihood, had much more upper body strength than I did. It wasn't that they almost got it either. None of those who tried seem to move off the floor at all. It made the video look all that much more impressive!

Then came the exhortations for me to try it. Why would I try it? I had just watched a half dozen people fail to move from the floor, and I had two formerly dislocated, weak shoulders, and this looked like it took very strong shoulders to complete. If the kids who were half my weight couldn't do it, I surely couldn't do it. I decided that they had taken the step to expose their vulnerability to each other, so it was my turn to be humbled by failure. I got down on the floor, stretched out my arms and pushed up. I was not very stable, but to my surprise, I was able to lift myself off the floor. I was stunned! I was absolutely certain that I could not do it. What I found out was that this exercise uses your core muscles much more than your shoulders, and I had a pretty strong core.

Here's the crazy twist. If no one had urged me to try it, I would have gone home that evening as if it were like any other evening. I was so convinced that I couldn't do it that I wouldn't have even tried it at home in private. It made me think about what other things I have never tried because I have convinced myself I can't do them. Those things I'm convinced I don't need to try fall into two categories: 1) Things that are one time accomplishments, such as the Lalanne Pushup, and 2) Things that require patience, persistence and much work to accomplish. The one time things are not too difficult to try, but the long term projects require an investment of time. What if I try one of those things, investing all that time, and then fail? The answer has to be, "So what!"

If we go through life afraid to try new things, we may miss out on some great things. My grandfather became a great artist and musician after he retired. I remember thinking how sad it was that he didn't even know he had those talents until he was past his 65th birthday. The truth is that he was good enough to make a living at it if he had only known at an early age. What about you? Have you ventured outside of your comfort zone and tried some new things? Have you tried the things that could make your running better or more enjoyable? Are you ready to train for a marathon? What are you waiting for?

Going outside of your comfort zone is difficult. It is a choice between comfort and risk, known and unknown. It seems like a choice between success and failure. If you stick to what you know, you feel like you will succeed, but will you? Nehemiah had the choice to stay in a comfortable bed and remain a cupbearer, but Jerusalem needed him. Like my situation with the pushups, if no one had told him about the shape his people were in, he never would have had the chance to make such an impact for God. I'm sure he faced doubt. What if he went and he couldn't accomplish what he went for? It was a risk. But Nehemiah knew that God was with him and was letting Him direct his path. How about you? What is God asking you to do that is outside your comfort zone?

- *That race that looks impossible just might be easier than you think. Maybe it's time to reconsider.*

- *Don't wonder if you can do something. Try it. If you fail, so what?*

- *Is God asking you to do something you're not sure about?*

- *Is God sure about it?*

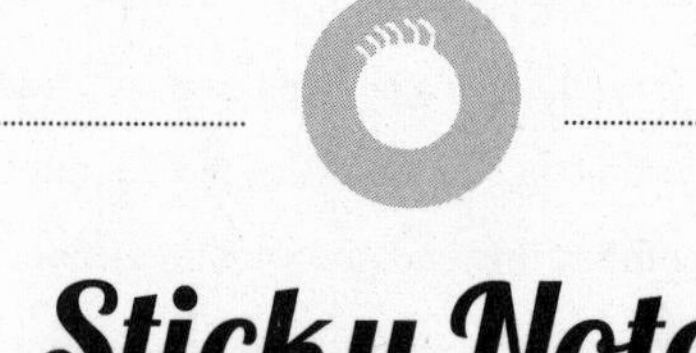

Sticky Notes

2
Week

my feet at his feet

I FOUND OUT IN FEBRUARY 2012 that I had high blood pressure. I also found out I had lumps in my throat. The surgeon said the word cancer about one hundred times in the brief five minutes he spent with me. I was so scared. He wanted to schedule surgery immediately. I needed to speak to an endocrinologist first since it was possibly thyroid related. Thank you God. God's direction took control; my fear of waiting too long didn't win over His direction. It wasn't cancer. It was lumps on my thyroid. The biopsy showed that they were all benign. PRAISE GOD! I decided to not look back, no more fear. I took control. I changed my eating habits and began a C25K program.

I completed the C25K program and ran my first 5k through Run for God. That first medal brought me to tears. I ran two more 5ks and really started to feel His presence in each and every step. I began a training program for a 10K next. It was tough, but I proceeded. I made it to the last week, which included one hour runs with no intervals. I WAS TERRIFIED. I did complete the first of three one hour runs. It was so hard. I felt fear creep in again. Will I have a heart attack? Will I fall and hurt myself?

I talked to many runners, hoping they would support me in my decision to not complete the last two one hour runs. Nobody backed me. I was going to give up and not graduate the program. When the morning came for my next one hour run, I got up, got dressed to workout, shut the bathroom door, and got on my knees. My fear was so overwhelming that there was no way I could even take the first step of that run. As I knelt before God in sincerity, it was as if God were sitting in the room with me on the edge of the tub with His mighty loving hand on my shoulder. I prayed, "God, you know me and You know my heart. I'm scared. You did not give me that spirit. Please take this run from me. I'll start running. You will be there. Thank you God."

That morning I had my best run to date. Every minute of that hour I felt more empowered. I smiled and teared up, too, as the clock ticked off the last 60 seconds. I completed the last one hour run two days later on the anniversary of 9/11. I kept 9/11 in my mind as I ran, thinking of what all of those poor people and their families had been through. The hour flew by. I was humbled by another's pain - my pain felt insignificant. God showed me a pain much, much, MUCH bigger than my own on the anniversary of that fateful day.

I completed and graduated the program. I am now signed up to run the Enchanted 10K with my lovely daughter, Lindsay, in February. I am currently running 5ks three times a week, and it feels so good. My running partner, my Heavenly Father, is always by my side. Truly, turn your life over to Him. Truly, believe that you have. Truly, trust God.

I am 52 years old. I have lost 60 pounds since this all began on that scary day in February 2012. I still have 25 pounds to go, and still am working to get off my blood pressure medicine - and I will. My God is showing me the way. The best things are built over time, and they all are built on lessons in trusting Him, letting go, having true faith, and never forgetting to say thank you God in advance of your success. Thank God in advance for His blessings on you today.

Caroline Murray – *Coral Springs, FL*

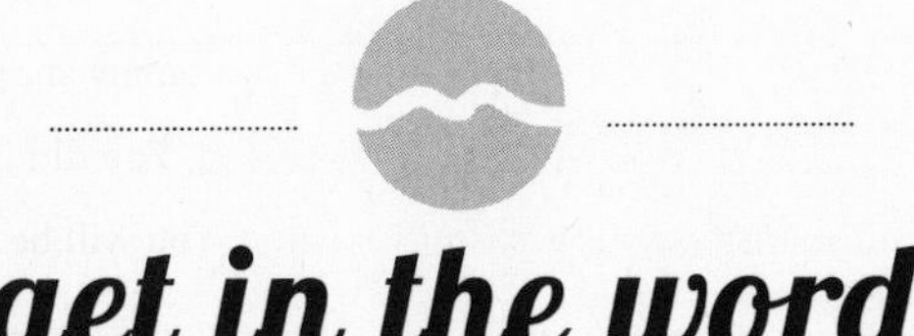

get in the word

Hebrews 12:1

Therefore we also, since we are surrounded by so great a cloud of witnesses, let us lay aside every weight, and the sin which so easily ensnares us, and let us run with endurance the race that is set before us.

Philippians 4:13

I can do all things through Christ who strengthens me.

2 Timothy 1:7

For God has not given us a spirit of fear, but of power and of love and of a sound mind.

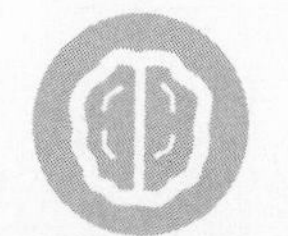

scripture memorization

Write out the scripture(s) in the space below and recite them ten times.

____

____

____

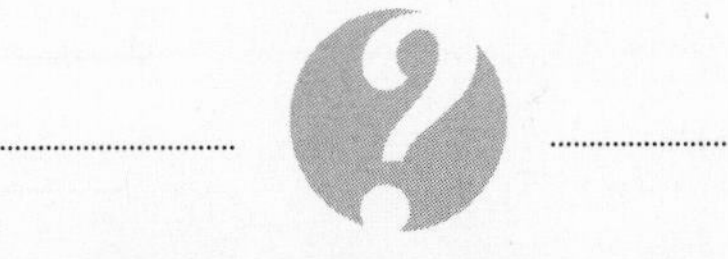

something to ponder

IS IT MY FEAR HOLDING ME back from pushing harder, and if so, why don't I truly believe that God is in control?

AM I WILLING TO LAY IT at His feet and let go?

DO I BELIEVE HE KNOWS MY heart, and knows that I HAVE DONE ALL I CAN IN THIS SITUATION?

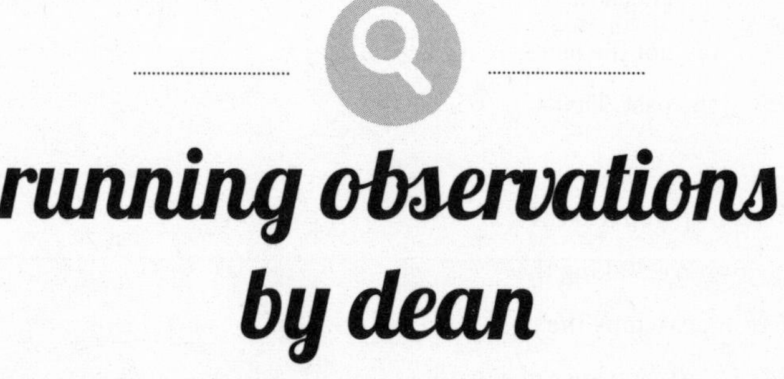

running observations by dean

When the Alarm Sounds

THE ALARM SOUNDS. IT'S TIME TO get out of the warm bed and go for a run on a harsh, cold, early morning. The voice in your head tells you to go back to sleep, hit the snooze button, roll over and sleep a little longer. Better yet, just reset the alarm and skip the run altogether. Everything in your body is telling you not to get up. You can make it up later. But you, warrior, throw back the covers in defiance of those voices in your head!

The weatherman said it may be raining in the morning, a ready-made excuse to skip the run. Checking outside, it's not raining, but it is a few degrees colder than the weatherman predicted. It sure is warm in the house, the voice says. You go to the kitchen, the voice getting louder, as you drink some water. Looking out the kitchen window, it looks like it could rain, though it is difficult to tell because it's still dark. You open the door to feel the temperature in order to dress appropriately, smells like rain.

As you walk to the closet to change clothes, there is still time to crawl back into bed and get some more rest. You battle with the voice in your head retorting with the thought that it will feel so much better and your entire day will flow like rain on a freshly waxed car after you have completed your run. You dress for a cold, dark, possibly rainy morning and tie your shoes. Once again, the voice tells you that you can make it up later. There's no point in going out into a cold, dark rainy morning when you need the rest. You tell the voice that your positive thoughts are what control you, not the negative, self-defeating thoughts that you have regretted listening to in the past. That's it! You're going out the door because you're a fighter!

Opening the door, you feel the cool, wet smelling air and decide it's exhilarating rather than adverse. Taking the first few steps is sluggish, tight and stiff. One last time, you're approaching the point of no return. Are you sure you want to follow through with this? You answer the doubt with the affirmation that you are going to do what you know is best, and you will win this battle.

As you continue to run, to get warmer, everything loosens up and you begin to feel better, confirming that you made the right choice. The coolness of the air makes you feel alive as you glide through the streets. You finish the run, the rain held off, and it feels great! The voices have been defeated once again and you are pleased with yourself for talking yourself into it.

1 Peter 5:8-10 says. "Be sober, be vigilant; because your adversary the devil walks about like a roaring lion, seeking whom he may devour. 9 Resist him, steadfast in the faith, knowing that the same sufferings are experienced by your brotherhood in the world. 10 But may the God of all grace, who called us to His eternal glory by Christ Jesus, after you have suffered a while, perfect, establish, strengthen, and settle you." God tells us that we all have to battle the voices of negativity that are authored by none other than Satan himself. Notice that He doesn't tell us that we MAY have to battle those thoughts, but He tells us to prepare ourselves ahead

of time so that when we see, hear and feel them, we are ready for rebuttal. Make up your mind today that you are not going to listen to the self-defeating, negative thoughts in your head!

- *When it is time to run, we often don't feel like going. We have to make a choice at that point between being comfortable now and uncomfortable later, or being uncomfortable now in exchange for being more comfortable later.*

- *Fill your head with positive thoughts, and let them be so strong that they crowd out and overwhelm the negative thoughts.*

- *We know that Satan is out there trying to make our lives miserable. When we submit to negative thoughts, we let him win. By preparing for those intersections between good and evil ahead of time, we can be ready to win the battle.*

sticky notes

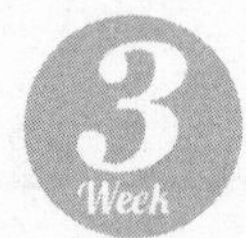

Elijah's run for God testimony

ELIJAH HAS A RUN FOR GOD testimony. He was calling all of Israel to turn away from their false god Baal and return to walk with the One True God, The Great I Am who had chosen them to be His treasured possession. He had this competition with the prophets of Baal to see which god was the mightiest. The prophets of Baal prepared a sacrifice unto Baal and cried out for him to set it afire. They shouted, danced, and even cut themselves with their spears and swords. Then it was Elijah's turn to show the Power of The One True God. He wanted everyone to know it was The Lord who set the sacrifice afire, so he poured water on the offering and the wood. He also poured the water in the trenches around the altar. He prayed The Lord would show Himself to all the people that they might KNOW there is only ONE True God. Fire fell and burned up the sacrifice, the wood, and licked up all the water in the trenches. There had been a drought that led to a great famine in the land. After this great show of the Lord's power, Elijah told Ahab to eat and drink for he could hear the sound of the heavy rains about to come down. Elijah sent his servant seven times to look for the rain he trusted and anticipated God to send. The seventh time, his servant sighted a small cloud rising from the sea. Elijah told his servant to tell Ahab to hitch up his chariot and go down before the rain comes.

Meanwhile, the sky grew black and the wind picked up, and a heavy rain fell as Ahab rode in his chariot to Jezreel. The spirit came upon Elijah and he began to RUN FOR GOD! He ran faster than the horses pulling Ahab's chariot. I imagine as he ran, tears were mixed in with these raindrops running down his face. I imagine each step he ran a little faster as he praised the Lord for all He had done that day. Elijah's prayers that his life would glorify the Lord were answered that day. He wanted his world to know that The One True God was Mighty. The Lord God had shown Himself strong that day. He sent down fire to consume the sacrifice placed on an altar soaked with water. The Fire of the Lord even licked up the water poured in the trenches.

Now it was raining. It was pouring. He was ending the drought and the famine with the downpour of rain. I bet He was counting his blessings as he ran. Don't you know he was singing in the rain as he ran "Bless the Lord, oh my soul... let everything that's in me Bless the Lord." Even his run glorified the Lord. He wouldn't have been able to outrun the chariot if the power of God had not enabled him. As I think upon Elijah's story, I want to do the same as he. I want to point others in my world to The One who bled and died to transform our lives. I want them to see God at work in me. I want to pray with expectation and always be on the lookout for God to "Reign" down an outpouring of His Spirit on my life. I want to RUN FOR GOD by His power at work within me.

Christy Hardy – *Northport, AL*

get in the word

1 Kings 18

And it came to pass after many days that the word of the Lord came to Elijah, in the third year, saying, "Go, present yourself to Ahab, and I will send rain on the earth." So Elijah went to present himself to Ahab; and there was a severe famine in Samaria. And Ahab had called Obadiah, who was in charge of his house. (Now Obadiah feared the Lord greatly. For so it was, while Jezebel massacred the prophets of the Lord, that Obadiah had taken one hundred prophets and hidden them, fifty to a cave, and had fed them with bread and water.) And Ahab had said to Obadiah, "Go into the land to all the springs of water and to all the brooks; perhaps we may find grass to keep the horses and mules alive, so that we will not have to kill any livestock." So they divided the land between them to explore it; Ahab went one way by himself, and Obadiah went another way by himself. Now as Obadiah was on his way, suddenly Elijah met him; and he recognized him, and fell on his face, and said, "Is that you, my lord Elijah?" And he answered him, "It is I. Go, tell your master, 'Elijah is here.'" So he said, "How have I sinned, that you are delivering your servant into the hand of Ahab, to kill me? As the Lord your God lives, there is no nation or kingdom where my master has not sent someone to hunt for you; and when they said, 'He is not here,' he took an oath from the kingdom or nation that they could not find you. And now you say, 'Go, tell your master, "Elijah is here"'! And it shall come to pass, as soon as I am gone from you, that the Spirit of the Lord will carry you to a place I do not know; so when I go and tell Ahab, and he cannot find you, he will kill me. But I your servant have feared the Lord from my youth. Was it not reported to my lord what I did when Jezebel killed the prophets of the Lord, how I hid one hundred men of the Lord's prophets, fifty to a cave, and fed them with bread and water? And now you say, 'Go, tell your master, "Elijah is here."' He will kill me!" Then Elijah said, "As the Lord of hosts lives, before whom I stand, I will surely present myself to him today." So Obadiah went to meet Ahab, and told him; and Ahab went to meet Elijah. Then it happened, when Ahab saw Elijah, Ahab said to him, "Is that you, O troubler of Israel?" And he answered, "I have not troubled Israel, but you and your father's house have, in that you have forsaken the commandments of the Lord and have followed the Baals. Now therefore, send and gather all Israel to me on Mount Carmel, the four hundred and fifty prophets of Baal, and the four hundred prophets of Asherah, who eat at Jezebel's table." So Ahab sent for all the children of Israel, and gathered the prophets together on Mount Carmel. And Elijah came to all the people, and said, "How long will you falter between two opinions? If the Lord is God, follow Him; but if Baal, follow him." But the people answered him not a word. Then Elijah said to the people, "I alone am left a prophet of the Lord; but Baal's prophets are four hundred and fifty men. Therefore let them give us two bulls; and let them choose one bull for themselves, cut it in pieces, and lay it on the wood, but put no fire under it; and I will prepare the other bull, and lay it on the wood, but put no fire under it. Then you call on the name of your gods, and I will call on the name of the Lord; and the God who answers by fire, He is God." So all the people answered and said, "It is well spoken." Now Elijah said to the prophets of Baal, "Choose one bull for yourselves and prepare it first, for you are many; and call on the name of your god, but put no fire under it."

So they took the bull, which was given them, and they prepared it, and called on the name of Baal from morning even till noon, saying, "O Baal, hear us!" But there was no voice; no one answered. Then they leaped about the altar, which they had made.
And so it was, at noon, that Elijah mocked them and said, "Cry aloud, for he is a god; either he is meditating, or he is busy, or he is on a journey, or perhaps he is sleeping and must be awakened." So they cried aloud, and cut themselves, as was their custom, with knives and lances, until the blood gushed out on them. And when midday was past, they prophesied until the time of the offering of the evening sacrifice. But there was no voice; no one answered, no one paid attention. Then Elijah said to all the people, "Come near to me." So all the people came near to him. And he repaired the altar of the Lord that was broken down. And Elijah took twelve stones, according to the number of the tribes of the sons of Jacob, to whom the word of the Lord had come, saying, "Israel shall be your name."[b] Then with the stones he built an altar in the name of the Lord; and he made a trench around the altar large enough to hold two seahs of seed. And he put the wood in order, cut the bull in pieces, and laid it on the wood, and said, "Fill four water pots with water, and pour it on the burnt sacrifice and on the wood." Then he said, "Do it a second time," and they did it a second time; and he said, "Do it a third time," and they did it a third time. So the water ran all around the altar; and he also filled the trench with water. And it came to pass, at the time of the offering of the evening sacrifice, that Elijah the prophet came near and said, "Lord God of Abraham, Isaac, and Israel, let it be known this day that You are God in Israel and I am Your servant, and that I have done all these things at Your word. Hear me, O Lord, hear me, that this people may know that You are the Lord God, and that You have turned their hearts back to You again." Then the fire of the Lord fell and consumed the burnt sacrifice, and the wood and the

stones and the dust, and it licked up the water that was in the trench. Now when all the people saw it, they fell on their faces; and they said, "The Lord, He is God! The Lord, He is God!" And Elijah said to them, "Seize the prophets of Baal! Do not let one of them escape!" So they seized them; and Elijah brought them down to the Brook Kishon and executed them there. Then Elijah said to Ahab, "Go up, eat and drink; for there is the sound of abundance of rain." So Ahab went up to eat and drink. And Elijah went up to the top of Carmel; then he bowed down on the ground, and put his face between his knees, and said to his servant, "Go up now, and look toward the sea. So he went up and looked, and said, "There is nothing." And seven times he said, "Go again." Then it came to pass the seventh time, that he said, "There is a cloud, as small as a man's hand, rising out of the sea!" So he said, "Go up, say to Ahab, 'Prepare your chariot, and go down before the rain stops you.'" Now it happened in the meantime that the sky became black with clouds and wind, and there was a heavy rain. So Ahab rode away and went to Jezreel. Then the hand of the Lord came upon Elijah; and he girded up his loins and ran ahead of Ahab to the entrance of Jezreel.

Malachi 3:10

Bring all the tithes into the storehouse, that there may be food in My house, and try Me now in this," says the Lord of hosts, "If I will not open for you the windows of heaven and pour out for you such blessing that there will not be room enough to receive it."

Ephesians 3:20-21

Now to Him who is able to do exceedingly abundantly above all that we ask or think, according to the power that works in us, to Him be glory in the church by Christ Jesus to all generations, forever and ever. Amen.

scripture memorization

Write out the scripture(s) in the space below and recite them ten times.

something to ponder

WHAT ARE you praying and expecting God to do in your life that will impact your world for Christ?

____

____

____

____

IN WHAT ways has the Lord opened up Heaven and poured out blessings on your life?

____

____

____

____

WHAT ARE YOU TRYING TO DO for the Lord that you cannot do unless His power is at work in you?

____

____

running observations by dean

What Were They Thinking?

Sometimes people are dishonest. Maybe they are reaching for something that makes them feel important. Maybe they are just trying to see what they can get away with. Whatever the reason, there are a few infamous occasions in the world of running. In general, the running community is an honest bunch, but every once in a while; there is a story that makes headlines when someone tries to cheat.

The most famous of these was Rosie Ruiz. She was crowned the winner of the 84th Boston Marathon in 1980 before it was discovered that she had not run the entire course. She had crossed the finish line in a time of 2:31:56, which was one of the fastest times ever at that point in history. There were a few problems that were apparent right away. First, she didn't seem very tired for someone who had just run a marathon. She claimed, "I got up with a lot of energy this morning." Second, she didn't look as lean as those who normally win marathons. Third, she had improved her time by over twenty-five minutes from her qualifying time, which she claimed to have run at the New York City Marathon. It turned out, after investigating, that she never even ran the entire New York City Marathon, either!

But that was years ago. There is no way anyone could get away with something like that today, right? Let's go to 2011, when Rob Sloan decided he was too tired to continue at 20 miles of the Kielder Marathon and took a bus to the finish line, coming in third place overall. At first, he claimed he had run the entire race, but let go of his claim after an investigation. The real third place finisher knew he had been third the entire race and was surprised when he crossed the finish line and was told he was fourth. He reported his suspicion and eventually was awarded third place. After learning that Mr. Sloan flagged down the spectator bus to catch a ride to the finish line, a "World's Dumbest..." title couldn't be far behind!

Then there was the case of Jason Scotland-Williams in 2014 who claimed to have run the second half of the London Marathon faster than the winner. The catch was that he ran the first half in 2:07 and then he ran the second half in 1:01. It turns out that he cut out about 9 miles of running as he cut across a barrier and joined the race further up. There were no split times recorded for him after halfway until 40km. It turns out, he ran the last 2k at about the same pace he ran the first 13 miles. Suspicious? I would say so. Incredibly, when he was confronted with the facts and eyewitness accounts of him going through barriers, he continued to claim that he just felt really good and he really did run that fast. He was eventually worn down and admitted to the ruse.

Why talk about cheaters? Because there are no shortcuts. If you want to get into great shape, it will take a lot of work. If you want to be competitively successful, you have to pay your dues. In addition, some people have such a need to "be somebody" that they resort to these things. When we have Jesus, we already know we're somebody. When it comes to spending eternity in heaven, the ONLY way you can get there is by shortcut! Jesus paid the price for us. We can't work hard enough to justify our spot in the kingdom. What Jesus did for me is not really fair. I get the grand prize and the race isn't even over! I wouldn't call it cheating, but when I think about it that way, it helps me to understand just how unworthy I am.

- *There have been several attempts at "cutting the course" and reaping benefits. What were they thinking?*

- *Whatever your running goals are, there are no shortcuts to get there. It takes daily, intentional work to get there.*

- *Jesus has made a way for us to take the express lane to heaven. We can't work hard enough to get there on our own!*

sticky notes

4 Week

get out of the boat

THE SUN WAS SETTING OVER THE calm waters of Lake Arrowhead in Luray, Virginia, on a warm summer evening. The next morning the waters would stir with hundreds of triathletes, all swimming to the buoys and completing the swim course. I was one of those triathletes that weekend; however, this triathlon would forever be etched in my mind.

I had completed triathlons before, but like all triathletes, the swim portion is always the most stressful. I was not a strong swimmer. In fact, I had grown to depend on my wetsuit for buoyancy and security in the water. This would all change this weekend. The water temperature of the lake was above 83 degrees, and due to safety concerns of overheating, the officials announced that wetsuits were not allowed, so I had a decision to make: swim without the wetsuit or withdraw.

I stood on the banks of the lake on Friday evening, pondering that decision. Standing beside me was a married couple, friends of mine, who were unbelievers. I was wearing a t-shirt, which had the scripture of Philippians 4:13 printed on the back, "I can do all things through Christ who strengthens me." As I was discussing my concern over the swim portion of this race, the wife walked over and put her hand on my shoulder, looked at the back of my shirt, then looked me dead in the eye and said, "I guess tomorrow morning we will find out if you believe what is written on your shirt."

I know what you're thinking, and your right. She called me out! I'm happy to say, when the horn blew Saturday morning, I entered the water without a wetsuit. The

Lord chose to strengthen my faith through an unbeliever, a t-shirt, and a body of water. The next time you lace up your shoes, ride your bike, or enter the water, will you be ready if God calls you out of the boat?

Thomas Daniel – *Verona, VA*

get in the word

Philippians 4:13
I can do all things through Christ who strengthens me.

Matthew 14:27
But immediately Jesus spoke to them, saying, "Be of good cheer! It is I; do not be afraid."

Matthew 14:31
And immediately Jesus stretched out His hand and caught him, and said to him, "O you of little faith, why did you doubt?"

scripture memorization

Write out the scripture(s) in the space below and recite them ten times.

something to ponder

DO YOUR actions match your faith?

WILL YOU be ready when your faith is tested?

SHOULD WE be content with our spiritual walk?

running observations by dean

We're Running Billboards

HAVE YOU EVER THOUGHT ABOUT HOW much information you carry with you as you run? I don't mean what's contained in your cell phone, if you happen to take that with you on runs. What's on your shirt? Many of us wear shirts we have accumulated from races. It typically includes the name of the race which occasionally includes the main sponsor, along with many other sponsors, as well as the charity the race benefits. That's a lot of advertising! But they earned that sponsorship. Whether they paid for a place on the shirt, donated food or other items, or participated in the event itself, races would be more expensive without those sponsors. The least we can do is support them by wearing the shirt, or shopping at the store, or using the service represented!

It doesn't stop there. We have logos all over our clothing. Some of us prefer a particular brand of shorts or tights, and we display that brand as we run. Allegiance to a brand is completely understandable because they all seem to fit and feel a little different. Some of us have odd body shapes and some brands fit us better than others. Some have luxurious feeling fabrics or breathe better. Whatever your motivation to prefer a certain brand over the many choices, you will be displaying free advertisement for that company for the life of the product. And that's perfectly okay with us, isn't it? Of course, almost everything you purchase today has a brand on it.

If you're like me, you look at people's shoes. There's no more talked about brand among runners than what we wear on our feet. If you search for it, you can find out what types of shoes the top several hundred runners at the Boston Marathon wore at this year's race. It's so important to us that we have people counting shoes on the course! If you ask a runner about her shoes, she will usually be happy to share all the details about them. We love our shoes!

The word brand comes from the Old Norse term "brandr" meaning "to burn." The human race has been branding for over 3,000 years and it became a marketing tool to brand packaging during the industrial revolution of the 19th century. Companies have been inventing more ways to get their product name or company name into public ever since. When you drive down the road, you will often see billboards and large marquees as you travel. The boxes you receive in the mail have the company imprinted on them. They don't want to miss a chance to advertise to the mail carrier! Brands and logos are everywhere!

What about us? Besides the clothing that we wear, what signs do we show through the expressions on our face? Can someone look at us and see who we are? Do we show the love of Jesus to those around us? Will others know who we are based on the fact that we are kind, moral, and good people? It's admirable if everyone around us knows what good people we are, but that's not enough. The Bible tells us that no one is without sin: "For all have sinned and fall short of the glory of God." Being good people who treat others with love and respect is the right thing to do, but it doesn't necessarily separate us from others. Christians do not have a monopoly on being good. You could be an atheist and be good to people. What separates us from others is what we do with The Great Commission. Jesus told us to share Him with the world. Although we can display a beautiful billboard that shows others we care, it is through our words that we distinguish ourselves as children of the king.

- *We're running billboards displaying logos and company names all over our clothes, shoes, and gadgets.*

- *Branding has been going on for a long time and continues to evolve. Today, even buildings are named for companies.*

- *What would happen if we expanded our reach, as Christians, in as many creative ways that marketing professionals have?*

March 3rd 2016 is a race/walk for 3miles at Kim Park - My Goal is to walk in that race - PS 19:5
Which is as a bridegroom coming out of his chamber, and rejoiceth as a strong man to run a race
I will rejoice as I look toward and prepare for this race

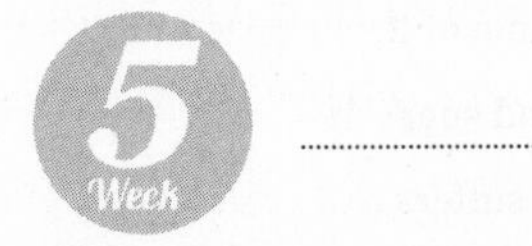

find me for yourself.

A FEW YEARS AGO, I WAS at a "plateau" in life -- nothing too stressful and nothing too exciting. I felt like God was a part of my life, but He was not leading me or really active in it. The unfortunate thing was that I was active in my church. As I was driving to work one day, I listened to What Do I Know of Holy, by Addison Road and I heard a voice say, "You've always been told where to find Me, now find Me for yourself." Then, it hit me. I no longer was pursuing a relationship with God. Fast forward a few months later.

I got married outside of the Catholic Church, which does not ensure job security when you work at your place of worship. I entered a second marriage without the proper process, and I was facing the loss of my job and my faith home. When this happened, I lost my ministry, my church home, many friends, and nearly every source of strength and sense of the presence of God. In addition, one place where I was able to recover and find my faith restored, a retreat center outside of Estes Park Colorado, was burned to the ground by a devastating fire. I looked for answers in the Bible and in my own way, I made a deal with God. I would read the Bible cover to cover, and when I was done, He would restore me to a ministry and I would find Him again. The thing with making deals with God is that most of the time I'm the only one in on the deal. When I got to the scriptures of the Babylonian exile, I realized we had something in common. I had been finding God in a place and so had they. God allowed that comfortable place to be taken away, so I could find Him in everything.

As I went through a time of depression and hopelessness, I couldn't seem to find God anywhere. A friend suggested that I get outside and get some fresh air every day. As someone who suffers from fibromyalgia, a good walk seemed like a good idea, and I knew I needed to find something to get me out of bed and out of the house. So the walks eventually turned into runs, and in those runs, I rediscovered God in nature, in the people I encountered, in the music I listened to, in the strength I didn't have at the end of a run when He made me strong, and in the ability to let go and allow Him to lead me on different paths and different journeys.

I have been able to lead two groups through the Run for God curriculum and am so very blessed to be able to share my renewed, personal, passionate faith with people through a program that also helps them to become physically healthier people.

Lara Dyer – *Colorado Springs, CO*

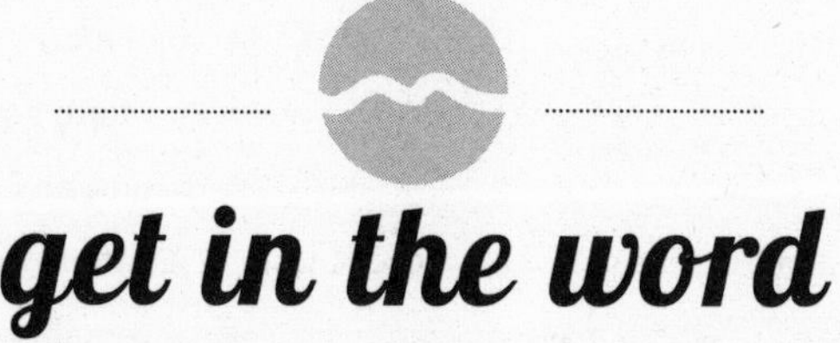

Isaiah 41:10

Fear not, for I am with you; be not dismayed, for I am your God. I will strengthen you,yes, I will help you, I will uphold you with My righteous right hand.

Matthew 12:22-31

Then one was brought to Him who was demon-possessed, blind and mute; and He healed him, so that the blind and mute man both spoke and saw. And all the multitudes were amazed and said, "Could this be the Son of David?"

Now when the Pharisees heard it they said, "This fellow does not cast out demons except by Beelzebub, the ruler of the demons."
But Jesus knew their thoughts, and said to them: "Every kingdom divided against itself is brought to desolation, and every city or house divided against itself will not stand. If Satan casts out Satan, he is divided against himself. How then will his kingdom stand? And if I cast out demons by Beelzebub, by whom do your sons cast them out? Therefore they shall be your judges. But if I cast out demons by the Spirit of God, surely the kingdom of God has come upon you. Or how can one enter a strong man's house and plunder his goods, unless he first binds the strong man? And then he will plunder his house. He who is not with Me is against Me, and he who does not gather with Me scatters abroad.

"Therefore I say to you, every sin and blasphemy will be forgiven men, but the blasphemy against the Spirit will not be forgiven men.

scripture memorization

Write out the scripture(s) in the space below and recite them ten times.

something to ponder

DO YOU strive every day to be in relationship with Christ?

HAS THERE EVER BEEN A TIME when you felt that God has called you out of your comfortable relationship with Him?

WHAT ARE the areas of your faith life in which you are too complacent?

running observations by dean

Runners Are Peculiar People

HAVE YOU EVER BEEN TO A runner's Expo? Most large races have them prior to race day. It's a chance for anyone who wants to get in front of a large number of runners to sell products or share a message to a captive audience. Usually, the runners have to go to the Expo to pick up their race packets and, of course, the path to those packets usually goes right through the vendors' booths. It is also a great time for runners to see all the latest gadgets, shoes, and nutritional products or to find a bargain on some older ones. Occasionally, we will set up a Run for God booth to share our story, hear others' stories and hopefully, connect runners to the best training partner anyone has ever had!

I like to watch people as they pass the booth and notice what a diverse and peculiar group we are. We come in every shape, size, and color. Some look fast and others, well, look less fast. Some come to wander around and see what they can find, while others are intent on getting what they came for and leaving the premises. Some come dressed as if they're ready to race and others come in business suits. Some are interested in what we have to offer, and some are not, but it's the nuances in their expressions that are most interesting.

We see a lot of runners who have never heard of us and they are elated about what we are doing. I can see their eyes light up as they settle on the Run for God logo and they rush to get closer. It's always exciting to see that expression and share our mission with them. It never gets old hearing how running and God has changed their lives for the better.

On the other extreme end of the spectrum, a few will show expressions of disgust. The Bible tells us that whenever we share Him, we will come against opposition.

The most interesting faces come from those in the middle of the spectrum when expressions are indifferent. In general, I find many runners to be confident people, and the idea of seeing something they don't believe in doesn't feel threatening to them, so they pass by seemingly unaffected. But, I have also noticed that there are times when I read that expression wrong. What looks like indifference and confidence is really just a front. Some of them change their expression as soon as I begin to talk to them, and those expressions are varied. They range from defiant, as if I am trying to indoctrinate them, to being interested in whatever I have to say. The defiant conversations are short, while the receptive runner discussions can be quite exhilarating. Although it looked like they were indifferent, I find that they are looking for something and sometimes it turns out that their answer is Jesus.

Although runners tend to be a little more focused and a bit high strung, there's one way that they are like everyone else. Everyone is looking for purpose in life. There are people around us every day, like those Expo attendees, who are waiting for someone to share with them. I am guilty of seeing the look of indifference on their faces and believing that they don't want to hear from me, but how many of them really want to hear what I have to share? There is only one way to know. Isn't it funny how God teaches us things in the places we don't expect and in ways we don't expect? I am not going to take those indifferent looks at face value anymore. How about you?

- *Runners' Expos are a great place to connect with runners of all types.*

- *The expressions on runner's faces as they walk through the Expo often say a lot about how they feel, but sometimes it is easy to misread those expressions.*

- *How many people around us are just waiting for someone to share Jesus with them?*

sticky notes

i am not a quitter

IN THE WINTER OF 2011, I started a couch to 5k program with a friend who lives in Chicago. Our plan was to train on our own then we would meet up in Chicago that summer to run a race together. It didn't go well. I started off great, then my friend got hurt, and it wasn't long after that I fell off the wagon; another attempt to get into a healthy routine, only to quit again. A few months later, I read in our church newsletter about a group that was forming where individuals could train to run a 5k; it was called Run for God. Most people would consider coincidence a factor with the timing of my quitting another "get healthy plan" and seeing a Christ-centered running group for women.

I had only been attending this church for a little more than a year when I joined this small group. Honestly, it took some time for me to see the hand of God in my life. When I started I could not even run for 90 seconds. As the weeks progressed I knew first-hand what one of my favorite running quotes truly meant. "It doesn't get easier, you just get better." I kept telling myself when race day came that if I could run half the distance and walk the other half it would be a victory. I ran the entire 5k at that October race in Detroit and was hooked. Our Run for God group is a women's only small group, and the friendships and camaraderie that have developed go beyond any experience I've ever known. I truly believe that putting God at the center is the key. I am not the fastest runner, but I have finished every race that I have entered. In April of 2012, several ladies from our group traveled to Dalton, Georgia to the "Run at the Mill" for our first half marathon.

I have run races all over Michigan and have completed races in Canada, Iowa, Pennsylvania, Tennessee and Georgia for the second time. In late 2012, I decided that it would be amazing to celebrate my 50th birthday on October 1, 2013 running the Detroit Free Press Marathon, the same event where I ran my first 5k two years before. I ran that race, not only with my Run for God sisters, but also ran with over 1000 runners from my church running for Hope Water Project. Each runner was challenged to run the marathon and each raise $1000 so that collectively we would raise $1 million to drill wells for the Pokot tribe in Northern Kenya, Africa. I reached my fundraising goal on my birthday, surpassed it in the end, and our team raised just over $1.3 million. In all of my 50 years, I have never relied on God like I did while I was training for and running that marathon. He was right there with me every step of the way, right down to my bib number. I went on the race website to get my bib number for packet pickup and many of my fellow church team members were posting their numbers on Facebook. I posted mine not realizing the significance until my friend Sherri's comment. Remember my reason for running this marathon, as a celebration of my 50th birthday on October 1, 2013? My bib number was "5013."

Since that first race in 2011, I have finished 53 races, including thirty-nine 5ks, two 8ks, one 7 miler, five 10ks, four half marathons, eleven 25ks, and one marathon. Even with all of those races and knowing that God is always with me, I still have struggles. It can be hard to get out the door for a run, and there are times when I feel lazy, fat and depressed, but I am not a quitter. I still run, and I'm still on the journey to be a healthier version of me, but I know that even though I am a work in progress, I can do anything with Christ. In most races, I am at the back of the pack and have always thought, too, that it doesn't matter if I come in last because my goal is always to finish. A few times, volunteers have commented on the fact that there were two or three people behind me. My comment was that it might happen, that I would be last, but it would not be that day. Secretly though, I never wanted the attention of being last. That changed with my second Run at the Mill in 2014. I knew all about the rolling hills of Georgia, but was undertrained due to our harsh

Michigan winter and getting sick weeks before the race. This would be my toughest half marathon and my first last place finish. The feelings that I thought I would have were not there. My dear friend, Rebecca, was with me for the entire race---she never left me, even when I begged her to go on without me. As we got to the last mile, the Run for God Junior Triathlon team came out to run with us to the finish line. Amid tears and cheers from the crowd and the five other "Crazy Michigan Girls" who made this trip, it was one of the best finishes ever.

God has blessed me with some pretty amazing finishes, like at mile 24.5 of the marathon. I was so tired and thought I had lost a toenail in my shoe. I also had some serious pain in the heel of the other foot. I kept praying for God to send His angels to help me lift my feet. I looked up and saw two hot pink Run for God sweatshirts. When the last sweeper bus came to the finish line and my running partners Rebecca, Jessica and I were not on it, Katherine and Leslie started walking the course backward to find us. I prayed for help to lift my feet, but they lifted our spirits and helped us to the finish line. With each milestone race, I added the Run for God distance sticker to my car. When I added the 26.2 and posted a picture, Mitchell Hollis made the comment that there were two more.

My friends know that it doesn't take much to plant the seed of an idea in me. Part of the reason that I have done so many races is because of my friend Katherine, who also ran her first marathon to celebrate her 50th birthday in April 2013. She suggested that "it would be fun" to run 26 races in the year of our marathon. So we did. Mitchell might be happy to know that 2015 is the year of the TRI and 2016 will be ULTRA special. Taking that first step on a hot and humid July evening, I could not ever imagine what God had in store for me. Distances I sometimes still can't believe that I've covered, the people I have met, the new friends I have made and the old friendships renewed are evidence of God's faithfulness. There is one who knew where this path would lead me and I am eternally blessed by running for Him.

Andrea Younkins – *Marine City, MI*

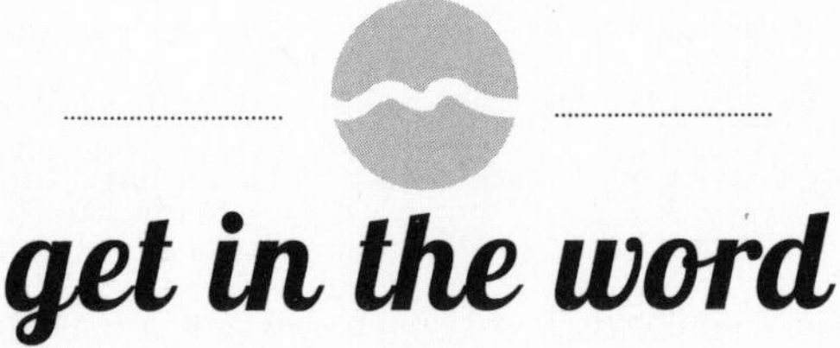

get in the word

Philippians 4:13

I can do all things through Christ who strengthens me.

Jeremiah 29:11

For I know the thoughts that I think toward you, says the Lord, thoughts of peace and not of evil, to give you a future and a hope.

Isaiah 40:31

But those who wait on the Lord shall renew their strength; they shall mount up with wings like eagles, they shall run and not be weary, they shall walk and not faint.

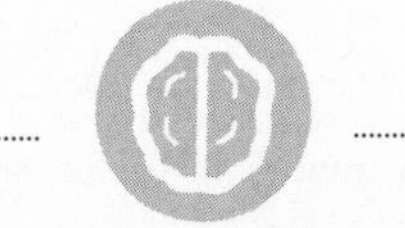

scripture memorization

Write out the scripture(s) in the space below and recite them ten times.

____

____

____

something to ponder

LOOKING BACK, can you think of a time when God's hand was clearly directing your path, but at the time you thought it coincidence?

I CHANGED the way I read Philippians 4:13. I used to emphasize I can do ALL things...but now read it as I CAN do all things. Can you name an instance where identifying with one word instead of another radically changed your thinking?

Like my angels at the end of the marathon, can you think of a time when you prayed for something and got an immediate response?

running observations by dean

Take Time to Enjoy Your Progress

RUNNING IS HARD WORK. IT REQUIRES sacrifice. There are a lot of other things to do, and many of them are much easier and more fun than running. It demands that we make time for it, and that investment of time is precious. The energy needed to be a runner can feel unattainable on occasion. There are moments when we wonder if it is all worth it. After all, it seems as if we just keep pushing the same buttons over and over again with the same results time after time. Once we are able to run twenty miles in a week, we push towards twenty-five. Once we are able to run under thirty minutes for a 5K, we have to push for twenty-eight. We're never satisfied. And that's good...if we keep it in perspective.

We didn't choose to be runners because we hate it. We have decided that it is the most beneficial form of exercise, both physically and mentally. Running fits well with our personalities and who we are. Sure, there are times when our relationship to running is one of love/hate. The blood, sweat and tears we shed feel good and bad at the same time. It's hard, but deep down, we really love it.

With all of that work, we are bound to make progress, but the world tells us that we should set a new goal once we reach an old one. There is a constant drive to achieve more, so much that we don't stop to think about what we have achieved. I think it is important to take the time to celebrate progress. It doesn't matter what your particular progress is, whether it is running twenty miles for the first time, losing ten pounds, or breaking twenty minutes for a 5K, stop for a minute to revel in your accomplishment. Everyone's progress is different and sometimes you have to dig to find something to commemorate, but there's always something, if you look hard enough. You may not feel like you are making progress, but you are! Think about how far you have come and not only about how far you have to go. Take time to celebrate!

There may be times when you have setbacks, such as an injury. It is easy to get down during these phases, but if you choose to change the way you look at your situation, you can find the good in it. For example, if you are injured and have to take a month off, just think about how much progress you will make in the first few weeks after you get back on your feet! Think about your successes and learn from the rough patches.

God established festivals and feasts. Jesus showed up at parties and weddings. God made us to celebrate! Colossians 3:15-17 says, "And let the peace of God rule in your hearts, to which also you were called in one body; and be thankful. Let the word of Christ dwell in you richly in all wisdom, teaching and admonishing one another in psalms and hymns and spiritual songs, singing with grace in your hearts to the Lord. And whatever you do in word or deed, do all in the name of the Lord Jesus, giving thanks to God the Father through Him." When good things happen to us, we should recognize them, and expressions of joy should spontaneously erupt!

- *We have a love/hate relationship with running.*
- *We should focus on not only how far we have to go to reach our goals, but also how far we come on our journey.*

- *God wants us to celebrate and give Him glory for our accomplishments. What can you celebrate and glorify God with today?*

sticky notes

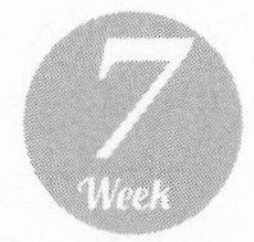

how i lost more when i surrendered it all

GROWING UP, I WAS NEVER ONE who struggled with weight. I was one of the thinnest in my group of friends. When I graduated from high school, I weighed 115 pounds which was much too light for my 5'6" frame. That all changed for me after I married and had four beautiful children. In my mind, I thought I could still eat like I did in high school. I soon found myself weighing over 200 pounds. I tried just about every diet I could. Many of them were not healthy. Of course, I would lose a few pounds at the beginning but quickly got bored and went right back to my old habits.

In May of 2013, I weighed 250 pounds. I was devastated. I finally realized I was trying to fix me by myself. I had surrendered my marriage and family to God, but I hadn't surrendered my diet. I prayed to God and told Him I was done fighting the battle alone. I laid it all at the cross. Shortly after this, I met a lady who had recently started going to a Run For God class in Joplin, Missouri. It sounded interesting, but I had NEVER been a runner. We started jogging together in the morning and she kept talking to me about the class. She was getting ready to graduate, but they were starting another group in a few weeks. I decided to join.

By the end of the 12 weeks, I had lost 45 pounds. God gave me the strength and resources I needed to get up off the couch and make a change for my family and myself. I am proud to say I have now lost a total of 60 pounds. I recently led my husband through his 12-week journey and we are gearing up to train for our first half marathon. God is so good! Don't be afraid to surrender it all to HIM. When we completely empty ourselves, the only thing left is for God to take complete control. At that time we experience complete FREEDOM!

Leona Belk – *Joplin, MO*

get in the word

Galatians 5:1
Stand fast therefore in the liberty by which Christ has made us free, and do not be entangled again with a yoke of bondage.

Psalm 37:23-24
The steps of a good man are ordered by the Lord, and He delights in his way. Though he fall, he shall not be utterly cast down; for the Lord upholds him with His hand

Mark 10:27
But Jesus looked at them and said, "With men it is impossible, but not with God; for with God all things are possible."

scripture memorization

Write out the scripture(s) in the space below and recite them ten times.

something to ponder

WHERE WOULD YOU BE IF YOU completely surrendered to God a year ago?

____

____

____

____

CAN YOU really get out of this mess on your own?

____

____

____

____

running observations by dean

Old Habits Die Hard

MAKING A PERMANENT CHANGE IS DIFFICULT for many of us. We get comfortable in our daily routine and flow through each day with little resistance, like a row boat floating down a river. Trying to go against the flow is hard. It takes a lot of effort. If we're really busy, the river is flowing fast, making it more difficult to change direction. For us older folks, our rudder is stuck in one position, and it takes great effort just to loosen it up to begin to go in another direction. The problem comes in realizing that great things will only come with purposeful change. That means work.

If you're trying to increase mileage, start cross training, eat better, or even begin running, it is going to be difficult. You have to change, and if you want to keep doing it, you will need to make that change permanent. I'm one of those who can begin something new, but I have trouble making it part of every day or week. Once the "new" wears off, it becomes difficult to motivate myself to get it done. I will slip back into my old routine rather quickly if I don't force myself to think differently. Over the past year, I began training for triathlons. I find it difficult to make myself bike, and even more difficult to swim. Riding takes a lot of time, so I have to schedule it as part of my day. Swimming is tough for two reasons: 1) I have to go somewhere to do it, and 2) I don't enjoy it. This is how I keep myself accountable: I make a commitment to myself at the beginning of the week that I will get in two rides, one of at least 20 miles and one of at least 35 miles, and two swims before the end of the week. I keep a log, so the lack of entries for riding or swimming will be obvious and will serve to motivate me the following week.

There is a different method that works for each of us, and trying to find what makes us focus on the change of habit can be difficult. In most cases, our days are already full. If we want to add something to the schedule, we have to give up something else, maybe a habit that is not so helpful. Trying to undo a more destructive habit, like watching too much television, is hard. The old saying "Old habits die hard" rings true every time we try to change something that we have been doing for years, but it can be done. A quote from British entrepreneur Charlotte Fantelli reads, "The easiest things are rarely rewarding. The rewarding things are rarely easy." If it were easy, most people would give up bad habits. But, it was Albert Einstein who defined insanity as doing the same thing over and over and expecting different results. If we don't change, we won't change.

God wants us to change. He expects us to change, every day. God says through Paul in Romans 12:2, "And do not be conformed to this world, but be transformed by the renewing of your mind, that you may prove what is that good and acceptable and perfect will of God." It is a constant battle to live apart from the world while living in the world. It takes persistent effort of constant change. The Bible tells us that we are not perfect, so we are to always be trying to improve our relationship with Christ, and that only happens with making regular changes to our lives and our habits.

- *It is difficult to change habits.*
- *If we don't change, we won't change.*
- *God expects us to change, daily.*

sticky notes

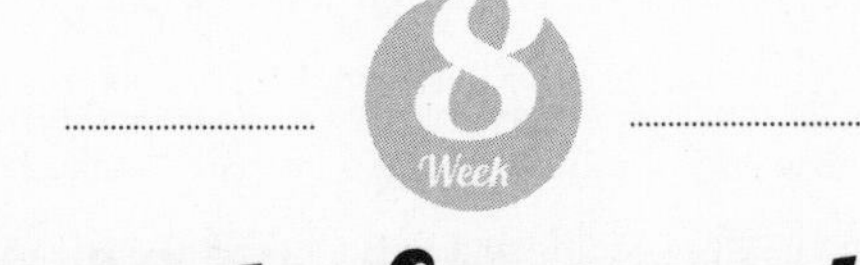

beauty from ashes

The pain was unyielding. Day after day I watched as my husband suffered through some of the most extreme headache pain imaginable. The viral meningitis he had contracted from a mosquito bite enflamed the lining around his brain, causing it to swell. Voices in his hospital room could be no louder than a whisper as even the high doses of pain medicine pumping into his body barely touched the swelling that pulsed in his head.

Each day that passed was a day that he slipped farther away from me, from reality. Here lay my best friend, in a hospital bed, suffering, unable to carry on conversation; I sat on the side of his bed, gently rubbing the side of his head with a warm cloth. I felt so utterly alone, so utterly helpless. Tears streamed down my face in the darkness of the room. My cell phone on vibrate; I saw the screen light up as multiple text messages arrived from friends and family members. I had no strength left to respond to their inquiries this night. Feeling my composure seeping away, I stole away to his small private bathroom. Crumbling to my knees on the hard tile floor, my world collapsed around me. The cries emanated from the bottom of my heart. "Yahweh, Yahweh, Yahweh!" As sudden as I took the next breath, sucking the air through my lungs, He arrived. Warmth wrapped itself around my shoulders and weaved through my soul. The most wonderful, comforting embrace I had ever felt. "There you are", I whispered. Never doubting the rivers of his mercy and comfort would arrive at my weakest moment, I welcomed Him with open arms. Faith assured me that even though I may be walking through this wilderness of sickness and disease, I would never walk it alone. The strength I was given that evening would be needed tenfold in the days and weeks and months to come.

After fighting through days of the viral meningitis, my husband's state of clarity and consciousness became fewer and further between. Worried expressions from nurses who entered his room every few hours concerned me as I watched them come and go. Over a week after he had been admitted to the hospital, instead of getting better, things only seemed to be getting worse. Then the day arrived. The day where the strength of the Holy Spirit was the only power moving my hands and feet forward. My husband had become almost completely unresponsive and was unable to move any part of his body from the waist down. Hurried motions and hushed whispers became a blur to me as I listened to a voice speaking from somewhere above me. A code was being called on my husband and the immediate transfer to the Neuro-Trauma Intensive Care Unit had begun. Tests were run; a myriad of questions were asked. A breathing machine was hooked up to his face to help assist his lungs, as he was unable to breathe fully on his own while he was sleeping. The doctors determined the viral meningitis had passed, but uncertainty lay around what might be causing the lower-body paralysis. As each day passed, I clung desperately to my Savior and to the promise that He would lead us through this storm in our lives. Finally, the day came where we had an official diagnosis. My husband had contracted Guillain-Barre, which is a disease contracted after an encounter with a viral infection. This disease attacks the nerves in your body beginning from your feet and working its way upward, causing temporary paralysis. Stopping at his waist, we were blessed that his upper body was spared from being paralyzed.

Thankful for the diagnosis, this was only the beginning. We were assured eventual recovery, but the process would be very, very slow. Standing in front of us were weeks of inpatient and outpatient physical therapy, nerve pain that was unlike anything either of us knew existed and emotional rollercoasters that at times threatened to throw us off the tracks of our faith. The one constant through our storm, despite the attempts to derail us from holding on to the hope and joy that were promised to us, was our Lord and Savior, Jesus Christ. Each day I woke up and prayed to be filled anew with the strength given to me by the Holy Spirit that night in my husband's hospital room. As I watched my husband heal slowly day-by-day, I remained ever humble and in awe of the merciful and unfailing love of Jesus. That very love enabled us to weather the storms around us and in doing so we are able to share that love and the healing power of God with those around us. The pain and fear that seized us in the beginning has now bloomed from the ashes into a beautiful masterpiece that could only be designed by the author of life himself.

get in the word

John 20:29

Jesus said to him, "Thomas, because you have seen Me, you have believed. Blessed are those who have not seen and yet have believed."

Romans 5:3-5

And not only that, but we also glory in tribulations, knowing that tribulation produces perseverance; and perseverance, character; and character, hope. 5 Now hope does not disappoint, because the love of God has been poured out in our hearts by the Holy Spirit who was given to us.

Psalm 30:8-12

I cried out to You, O Lord;
And to the Lord I made supplication:
"What profit is there in my blood,
When I go down to the pit?
Will the dust praise You?

Will it declare Your truth? Hear, O Lord, and have mercy on me; Lord, be my helper!"
You have turned for me my mourning into dancing; You have put off my sackcloth and clothed me with gladness, To the end that my glory may sing praise to You and not be silent.

O Lord my God, I will give thanks to You forever.

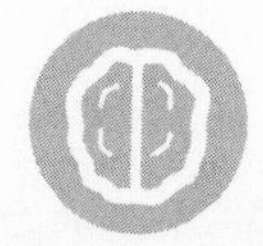

scripture memorization

Write out the scripture(s) in the space below and recite them ten times.

something to ponder

What is your initial coping mechanism when you experience a trial in your life?

WHAT MIGHT keep you from experiencing joy during a painful situation?

HOW MUCH more of an impact in the lives of others do you think we could be if we realized that God can use any situation for His glory?

____

____

____

____

running observations by dean

On the Course or Watching?

ANYONE WHO HAS EVER PARTICIPATED IN any sport knows how difficult it is to watch that sport, particularly if it is an event that you could be participating in, but can't because of an injury or other circumstance. The want and/or need to be out there in the middle of the action is overwhelming. Don't get me wrong, spectators are very important to any event, but sometimes it's hard to be a spectator. Another difficult time to be a spectator is when your child is participating and you want to help. Watching my oldest son, Matthew run a cross country race always made me want to get out there and run with him, to try to make it easier for him, to take away the pain, anything, just to help! Or when my youngest son, Caleb would be on the golf course, competing, and I knew I could hit the shot he needed to hit, but he might struggle with it. I wanted to take the club and swing it so badly! But, I couldn't do anything in either case. I had to leave it in their hands to do their best.

I remember, during my junior year of high school, having a case of tendonitis in my foot. I had to wear a cast for two weeks, and it happened that there was a big track invitational in Florida that I desperately wanted to run. I wanted to be there so bad that I rode down in the van with the guys who were going to run, but since I couldn't participate, I couldn't have my meals paid for by the school. So, I brought about fifteen peanut butter and jelly sandwiches with me so that I would have something to eat while everyone else was eating. They would go into a restaurant and I would take a couple of sandwiches in and eat with them. On the ride down, I remember wanting to bet everyone that I could still run a six minute mile with a cast on my foot. We were trying to figure out when I would be able to try it when the coach found out and put a stop to the attempt before I could try it. I wanted to participate so badly, that I was willing to stage my own event to make myself feel relevant. I didn't want to sit on the sidelines.

Again, having participated in hundreds of events in my lifetime, I can say with all confidence that spectators have often been a big performance booster. They are appreciated more than they know. And when the event I am watching is one where I cannot participate, it is much easier to watch. I don't want to minimize the role of the spectator in sporting events, especially running.

In life, I'm afraid we have spectators and we have participants. Some people are doing things and making things happen, while some are sitting on the sidelines. In some cases, the implications are small. But when it comes to salvation, the implications are huge. Not only do we need to make sure that we are full participants, we have a responsibility to sign others up for the race. It is a race where we don't want spectators. The only inspiration we need is Jesus waiting at the finish line. The encouragement comes from Him and our fellow participants in the race. He is all the reason we need to get off the couch!

- *Watching an event you want to participate in can be mentally tough.*

- *Watching your children participate in sports can be tough. Don't you think that is how God looks at us as we go through life?*

- *When it comes to salvation, we can't be spectators. We have to get off the couch and become full, all out participants, giving Him our absolute best!*

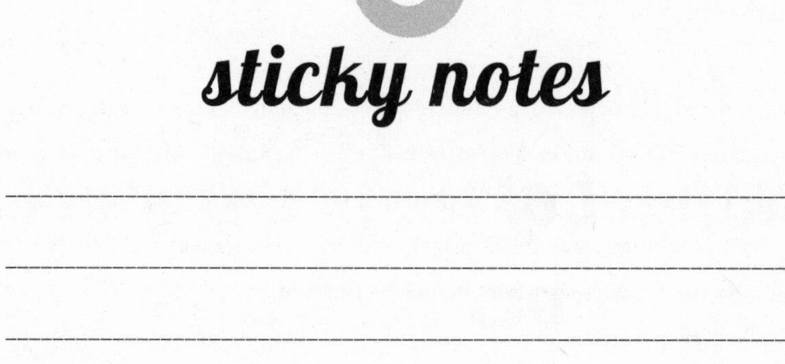

impact of a shirt, impact of our presence

WHEN WE STRIVE TO BE GOD'S hands and feet, I can't help but wonder sometimes what portion of our words or actions leave a lasting mark with those on the outside watching us. Some call it "the ripple effect" when the waves we make splash up on others. Sometimes we are blessed to see the impact of the waves, but many times we are left to wonder if they ever splashed up on anyone or anything.

Two years ago our first Run For God 5k class was presented with an opportunity to serve the hydration station at an area half-marathon race. Most in our group had never witnessed a race of that distance and were expecting to see a collection of elite athletes. Instead they saw an inspiring group of nearly 2,000 runners of all ages and abilities giving it their best to persevere, much like we were trying to do with our 5k training. Our goal had been to be witnesses for Christ as we served as His hands and feet to other runners that Sunday morning, and we were also blessed with it being a great fellowship opportunity with one another. Last year our 2nd class chose to serve that same race again. We asked to serve at the final hydration station just before mile 12 in the race to help provide participants with the motivation to make it to the end. Once again, we were inspired by the effort and courage of participants. Some stopped to pray with us, and so many commented on our Run For God shirts.

Toward the end of the race, I noticed a runner staggering through the station, and I knew he was in real trouble. As I stepped out to meet him, he quickly snapped with slurred speech, "You are not going to stop me, I am finishing this race!" He could not be convinced to rest even for a few minutes. As he continued to stagger and weave past our station, I pulled out the emergency number I had been given and dialed the number for the race organizers. Unfortunately, I did not get the man's bib number, all I had was a description of what he was wearing and the name printed on his bib, Tony. The race was another inspiring experience for our group, although I couldn't help but wonder what had happened to Tony. We prayed for him at our next class.

This past spring the same company that put on the half-marathon race approached our Run for God group about volunteering at the biggest half-marathon race in the state with 14,500 people. I gave it prayerful consideration, but decided not to do it since we had a large number that would be running in the event as the goal race for RFG Half-Marathon training. One of the employees for the race organizer happened to also be a past RFG instructor. She reached out to me with an opportunity to pass out shirts at the race expo rather than serve at a hydration station. It would provide the chance to reach each participant with ample time for conversation, but would require getting nearly 40 volunteers to serve over two weekdays. Our team committed to doing it as a way to reach more people on a more personal level.

In preparation for the expo, we created information cards to share with those who asked about our shirts and had those available at our tables. At the expo, it was a sight to see our group wearing their Run for God shirts, standing behind the tables and passing out the event shirts. Some runners commented that they wished we were handing out Run for God shirts rather than the race shirts. Our team split the expo hours into three 5-hour shifts over those two days. On each shift, some worked the packet table handing packets to participants, some worked the shirt table, a row behind the packet table, locating shirt sizes for the packet table, while others worked in the back stuffing race packets. I served on one of the shifts on the second day and was only at the packet table for about 20 minutes, but that's all God needed.

While I was standing at the table putting bib pins together in groups of four, a man in a business suit approached the table and pointed at the Run for God logo on my friend's shirt next to me. This man said "You guys saved my life." My friend wasn't sure what he meant, and the man went on to share, "Last summer your group served at a hydration station at the Emerald City Half Marathon. I was in bad shape at the final water stop and someone from your group called ahead to medical. They were waiting for me, and that saved my life." My friend instantly remembered the story from the previous summer's RFG 5K class about a man who was weaving and had refused to stop. My friend pointed to me and said, "Sir, I think this is the man that helped you." The man looked me in the eyes and started crying as he introduced himself as Tony and said, "Thank you." The world seemed to stop for those 5-10 seconds as we both cried. Out of 14,500 runners, out of three shifts working the packet table, and during the 20 minutes I was in that location, God reunited Tony and me, and it was a beautiful thing. That day was one of those occasions where God allowed for the splash of the ripples to be seen, a "God Moment." I can't help but wonder if God was smiling from above that day as he pushed Tony and I closer towards each other that day. That day validated for me once again the impact of this running ministry. Organizing and planning activities are no simple feat, but we just offer ourselves to God in faith that he will use us as he sees fit. That day validated for me the power of our shirts. Tony didn't recognize me, he recognized God's shirt. We were there on behalf of God, not as individuals. That day Tony also learned what Run For God was all about, he ended up taking two information cards.

Ben Reed – *Westerville, OH*

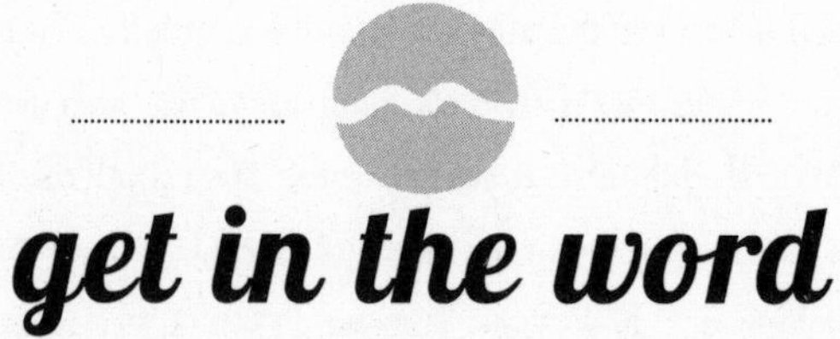

get in the word

Philippians 2:13

For it is God who works in you both to will and to do for His good pleasure.

John 14:12

"Most assuredly, I say to you, he who believes in Me, the works that I do he will do also; and greater works than these he will do, because I go to My Father.

2 Corinthians 5:20

Now then, we are ambassadors for Christ, as though God were pleading through us: we implore you on Christ's behalf, be reconciled to God.

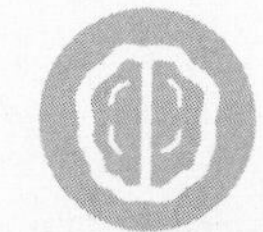

scripture memorization

Write out the scripture(s) in the space below and recite them ten times.

____

____

____

____

____

____

____

____

____

something to ponder

WHEN HAVE YOU OFFERED YOURSELF TO God and wondered if you have succeeded in doing His work?

WHERE HAS God blessed you in allowing you to see Him use you for His plan?

WHAT NEW ways can we offer ourselves for the glory of God?

running observations by dean

Ode to the Volunteer

LIKE MANY RUNNERS, I RUN A lot of races throughout the year. I run distances from a mile to a marathon, some hilly, some flat. I've run through downtown streets and country roads. I've participated in no frills races with no t-shirts or awards, just a line in the dirt, as well as mega-organized races like the Boston Marathon. There are endless choices of races to run with more diversity than Jeopardy has answers. Like the runners participating in these events, they come in all shapes and sizes, but there is one thing that all races have in common: If it were not for volunteers, the starter's pistol would never venture to fire.

For a typical race, I get up at 5:30 or 6:00 a.m. for an 8:00 a.m. start. It's tough to get up at that time on a Saturday morning, but some of the volunteers have been awake since 3:00 or 4:00 a.m. There is a lot to set up prior to my arrival. Not only that, some of them spent the entire day on Friday getting everything ready for Saturday. When I get to the race location at 7:00 a.m., the volunteers are there to greet me and give me what I need to be ready for the race and answer any questions I may have (and boy do they get some crazy questions). If I'm in a grumpy mood, it doesn't last long because they turn me around with their enthusiasm. Those volunteers are some happy people!

When I leave them still working for everyone else in the race, I have time to prepare for the race with my warm up. The volunteers are all around, directing traffic, parking cars, making sure everything is safe, and just being a general help to everyone arriving.

We are called to the starting line where we are given last minute race directions, maybe the National Anthem and a prayer, and instructions on what to do after we finish. They have so much faith, they EXPECT us to finish! Once the gun sounds and we are trying to get the most out of our bodies, volunteers along the course point the way, ensuring that we don't miss a turn. When we get thirsty, volunteers will hand us a cup of something to drink, often offering us a choice. For longer races, they even offer us some food to help with our journey.

When we finally arrive at the finish line, there are volunteers working hard to make sure our times are accurate when they are recorded. If there is a timing chip on your shoe, they will remove it so that you don't have to. They work feverishly, as everyone is finishing, organizing the results as fast as they can because they know everyone wants to go home as soon as possible.

From the finish line we walk to a table filled with food and drinks, placed there and maintained by volunteers, to ensure we get the best possible recovery. Some of us will run a cool down, while others will sit down and enjoy the food, often listening to some music or some other form of entertainment. Many races offer door prize drawings too! Those folks think of everything!

After the sustenance, it is time for the awards, which were designed, ordered, secured and brought to the race location, usually, by volunteers. The race director calls out names from the results tabulated from a race that only happened thirty minutes ago and hands out awards to the faster folks. They thank the sponsors and volunteers because they know there could not have been an event without them.

But they're not done. Many volunteers hang around for clean-up duty after the awards presentation and after all the runners have gone home. It is a thankless job to be sure, but one that must be done out of respect for the venue. When all this is completed, and the volunteers are ready to go home, they begin to talk about next year's race and how they can make it better than this year. They will do it all again, some in a few weeks or months and some in the following year's race, but there is one thing that I see in all volunteers; a servant attitude. Take time to thank volunteers at your next race. They work hard, and your kind words may be the only payment they receive.

Close to the end of the Sermon on the Mount, Jesus tells us in Matthew 7:12, “Therefore, whatever you want men to do to you, do also to them, for this is the Law and the Prophets.” Don’t you love it when someone lets you know that they appreciate what you do for them? Everyone likes to be recognized for being helpful. The volunteers at the races we attend deserve our gratitude for what they do. At your next race, take time to thank some volunteers. Your words are not the reason they do it, but they can be a tremendous blessing to someone who needs it.

- *Races would be nearly impossible to pull off without volunteers working long hours for no pay to ensure you have a great experience.*

- *There are many things that volunteers do that we take for granted. How would you like to be in charge of ordering port-a-potties?*

- *Jesus wants us to treat people the way we would want to be treated. With that in mind, take time to show true thankfulness to the volunteers at your next race.*

soul running - running with God

I STARTED RUNNING AT THE AGE of 39. I always hated running. It was my least favorite form of exercising until God asked me to go for a run. I didn't hear him audibly say it, but He did. He held out his hand and said it is time.

I went to a local boot camp to lose some weight that had been creeping on after having three kids and turning thirty. I started working out in a way that was beyond anything I had ever done before. Back "in the day," I played volleyball, but hated the running for conditioning. As a young adult I went through a phase of vigorous workouts, step classes, videos, aerobic kickboxing, but not running. However, God said "Let's go for a run." I was skeptical, but I went.

At first it was a half-mile then I would quit and walk. I knew I must look ridiculous. Then I found a running buddy and we made it to .80 miles. We still laugh about how "we used to have to stop at the stoplight to breathe." One mile turned to two, then to three miles. Soon we were meeting two to three mornings at 5:00 a.m. to run. We ran our first 5k in frigid temperatures, and it was awesome. It wasn't long before we made it to five and six miles. Then my buddy started training for a half marathon. I knew this was her goal, but God had something else in mind for me.

Running became soul searching for me. God would often reveal a truth to me about Himself during our runs. I was struggling with a lot of anxiety, and running gave me an escape. Then I realized it was not an escape from pain in my heart, but I was running a course towards the pain in my heart. In order to let the pain go, I had to face it. As a young preteen I lost a childhood friend due to tragic circumstances. While I always felt God wanted me to write about my story, I had not healed. I had buried the pain and guilt. When I was running, God was guiding me physically and spiritually to a place to lay it down. I sought counseling and was given a chance to speak at a ladies class and speak about the summer twenty-seven years ago that had changed me forever. I laid it down. Then I laid my dream down. Accepting that God's plans are better than mine and that if He wants me to write about it, He will make a way.

At the same time, I was struggling with a friend who was diagnosed with breast cancer, personal finances, anxiety and marital stress. Still I ran. Running taught me about consistency, challenging myself and staying the course, both physically and spiritually.

I have to train for a 5k, 10k and Warrior Dash. I have to train the same way in my daily spiritual battles. Running has taught me endurance. You have to want it to stay in it. Although I struggle with anxiety on a daily basis, I endure and persevere just like I do when I am running. I want to get better. I want victory. Without the challenge you can't have victory. I pray and pray some more. I run and run some more. Just like on my running path, if I fall down (which I have twice) I get back up, shake it off and keep going.

Now, we all know God's timing is perfect. During my friend's struggle with breast cancer, I was driving home one day, looking up at the sky. I prayed. She was extremely nervous about a bone scan she was about to have. The clouds were gigantic that day. I prayed to God to please let my friend be okay. I didn't even care if my husband and I lost our house. Her life was more important than the worries in my heart. About two weeks later I pulled into my driveway one afternoon. She called and gave me the news that she was cancer free. Five minutes later, I walked into my home of 10 years where I raised my children, and my husband told me our house was being foreclosed. When God gave me my friend's news, I knew he gave me exactly what I needed to increase my faith and to trust his plan for me. So I went for a run.

Hayley Barnes – *Hazelwood, MO*

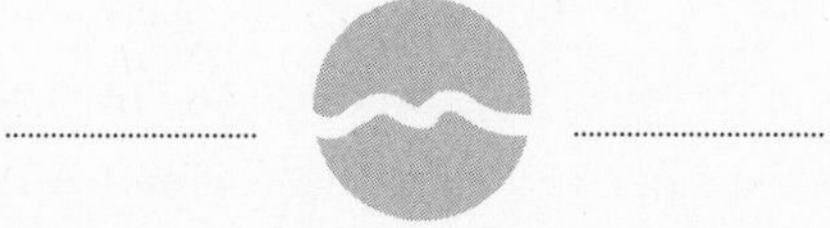

get in the word

Philippians 1:6

Being confident of this very thing, that He who has begun a good work in you will complete it until the day of Jesus Christ;

Matthew 21:22

And whatever things you ask in prayer, believing, you will receive."

Romans 5:3-5

And not only that, but we also glory in tribulations, knowing that tribulation produces perseverance; and perseverance, character; and character, hope. Now hope does not disappoint, because the love of God has been poured out in our hearts by the Holy Spirit who was given to us.

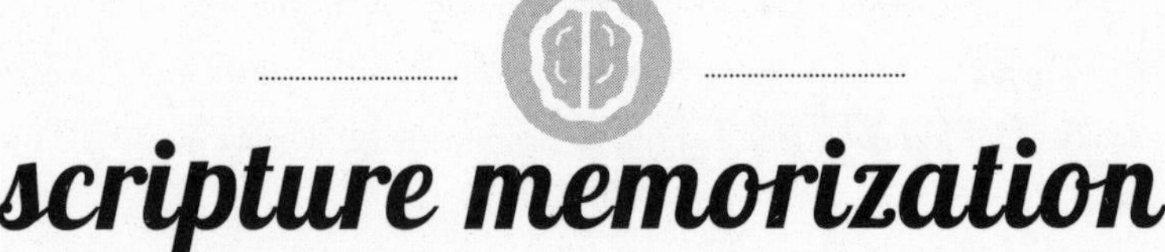

scripture memorization

Write out the scripture(s) in the space below and recite them ten times.

____

____

something to ponder

DO YOU trust God enough to give Him your dreams even if His plans are different?

HAVE YOU prayed big?

HAVE YOU been stuck in a season of stress or depression? If so, how did you endure?

running observations by dean

When Consistency is Not Good

CONSISTENCY IS A GREAT THING. IN order to be a runner, whatever your ability, you must train regularly to be as successful as you can be. Everyone's idea of success is different, but whether your goal is just to complete a half marathon or to qualify for the Boston Marathon, consistent training is integral to reaching your goal. If you run six days this week and then none next week, it is not the same as running three days a week. Consistent running is important, and many of the supporting activities for runners must be carried out consistently, too. For example, if you only eat healthy every other week, it's probably not doing you much good. While having a bad day may not affect you much, a full week will have an impact. If you focus on staying well hydrated at times, while ignoring it others, you're probably not going to get the most from yourself. It's the same for stretching, core-training, and any other supporting activity that you do to either keep you in shape or help your running.

On the other hand, can you get too much of a good thing? Can you eat too healthily? Probably not. Can you be too hydrated? You can, but it would take an awful lot of water. Can you stretch too much? No. You can run too much, but that's not the point I want to get to. There are times when we do too much, and it doesn't cause a physical problem. What do I mean by that? Motivation is an important factor in our running. Anyone who has ever run for more than a few months knows what it is like to struggle to find motivation to run. I believe the motivation issue is sometimes due to too much consistency. For example, if you run the same route every day and run it at the same pace every day, it's no wonder you get bored. In the same way, if you run the same workout every Tuesday evening, it will get old. Mix it up and be less consistent.

How about a deeper issue? If you always deny yourself dessert because you are so concerned about your diet, you may become resentful of the fact you always have to turn it down. That gets in the way of motivation. It goes the same for drinking water. The once every few months soft drink won't kill you. If you would rather not drink that soft drink or eat that dessert, it's probably not getting in the way of your motivation. If you're that person, great! But, for most of us, we struggle a little with denial. Don't miss the forest for the trees. Don't let the little things block your vision of the big picture.

God calls us to have consistent Bible study and prayer. You can't be a good runner without consistently running. You can't be close to God without a consistent connection to Him. Can we do too much? In most cases, no, but when we look at the Pharisees in the Bible we see religious leaders who were great at repetition and saying long prayers in public. But their purpose was only to follow rules and procedures and they completely missed the big picture. Their focus was on themselves and not on the needs of those around them. In today's world where we are all so busy, it's easy to lose sight of the neighbor who needs help. We may be going to church and be active while we're there, but if we miss the needs of those around us, we've missed the forest.

- *Consistency in your running and all the supporting activities is one of the most important variables to your success.*

- *Too much consistency can lead to a lack of motivation.*

- *God wants us to have a consistent relationship with Him instead of consistent repetition of rituals.*

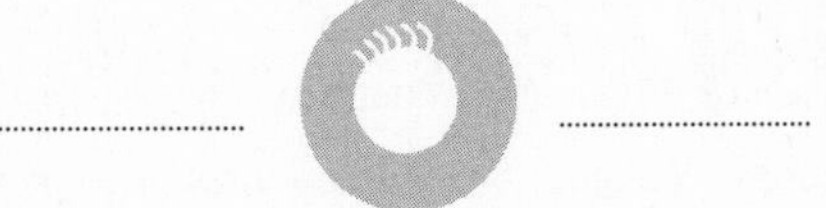

sticky notes

my boston story

WHEN I CROSSED THE FINISH LINE on April 15, 2013, I was so disappointed.

with my finish time. It was a lot slower than I had trained for and set for myself. Fifteen minutes later, everything changed. Disappointment turned to fear for my family, not knowing if they were okay. Once we were together, that fear turned to gratitude. As I walked the two and a half miles back to our motel surrounded by my family, I began to feel so guilty. Seeing the faces and hearing the crying of so many runners who were stopped within a few miles of finishing was heartbreaking. They had the same goals and dreams as I did, but were denied the opportunity to cross the finish line. Many were unsure of the well-being of their families because of a senseless act by two misguided young men.

How could I be disappointed when at least I was able to cross the finish line because of where I was in the wave lineup? Another example of God's hand in my life: He had provided me with the strength to qualify at Chickamauga with a time that put me in the next to last corral of wave 2. I didn't know at the time, but if I had run the same time in wave 3, I would have crossed right as the bombs went off. But still, how could I be happy when so many were suffering? I praise and thank God for His hand of protection over our family. When I hear of the recoveries and strength of the injured, I am inspired and it helps me deal with the rollercoaster of emotions that I still struggle with daily.

Isaiah 40:31 is special to me because I have read the stories of recovery and know from my own experiences that when we turn our burdens over to God, we can rest assured that He will give us the strength to get through them in His perfect time. When I look back today, I can see how God was preparing me for future events. You see, on February 24, 2014, our family lost everything, including 3 cats that were loved dearly, in a house fire. All we had were the clothes we were wearing and what was in our cars. Through God's grace and provision, our family of 5 pulled together. Friends and family flooded us with prayers and support. God's hand was in each and every obstacle that we faced. Today we have a new home, have adopted 2 shelter cats and are rebuilding our lives. I am so thankful for the opportunities that God has given us. To God be the glory and may we have faith and focus to finish the race God has set before us.

Virginia Brooks – *Hull, GA*

Psalms 73:26
My flesh and my heart fail; but God is the strength of my heart and my portion forever.

2 Thessalonians 3:3
But the Lord is faithful, who will establish you and guard you from the evil one.

Isaiah 40:31
But those who wait on the Lord shall renew their strength; they shall mount up with wings like [illegible] *they shall run and not be weary,they shall walk and not* [illegible]

scripture memorization

Write out the scripture(s) in the space below and recite them ten times.

____

____

something to ponder

HOW CAN we use the examples of Jesus to help us focus and finish the race that is set before us?

HOW CAN I use my personal experience to honor God and encourage others?

running observations by dean

Best Day of the Week

Is there a particular day of the week that is best to run? Let me try to make the case:

Monday is the best day of the week to run because it is a fresh start and an opportunity for you to fulfill a weekly goal. It's another opportunity to be the runner you want to be. If you run after work, it's a great way to unwind after the shock of going back to work. Getting in a good run is essential after gorging yourself on the weekend free-for-all at the buffet!

Tuesday is the best day of the week to run because you have had some rest since your weekend long run. Tuesday runs usually feel good. Studies show that Tuesday may be the best day to have surgery, so be thankful you're running and not having surgery!

Wednesday is the best day to run because it's hump day! It feels great to get in a good run in the middle of week, knowing that there are only a couple of days left until the weekend. And it's fun to pronounce the day in three syllables, Wed-nes-day. The word on the street is that Wednesday is the best day to get good deals at the grocery store. Some people run to eat, so it's a good day to celebrate.

Thursday is the best day to run because it's the penultimate day of the work week. It's the best day to reflect on the previous days of the work week as you take out your frustrations on the road or trail. It's time to plan your weekend agenda. The epiphany for a great weekend idea can come to you from the solace of a Thursday run.

Friday is the best day for running because...it's FRIDAY! If you're a high school football fan, it's game day. If you're a college football fan, you're thinking about game day. If you're a professional football fan, well, did I mention it's Friday!

Saturday is the best day to run because it's race day. If it's not race day, you can think about how many training weeks there are until race day. For many, it's long run day. Usually, Saturday mornings are not the same rush as every other morning of the week. It's a shame Saturday morning cartoons are not what they used to be, though.

Sunday is the best day to run because it's church day. It's also the day when the newspaper is extra fat with more stories and sales advertisements. Is there a sale on running gear?

- *Who am I trying to kid? The best day of the week to run is TODAY!*

1 Thessalonians 5:16 says, "Rejoice always, pray without ceasing, in everything give thanks; for this is the will of God in Christ Jesus for you." Give thanks to Him every day for giving you the ability and desire to take care of your body/temple. Use your running time to get closer to God. I find that He is an excellent listener even when I am running at a pretty fast clip. And He's not even breathing hard.

What is your favorite day of the week to run?

- *Find joy in every day that God gives us to run. Remember, this the day that the Lord has made.*

- *God tells us to be thankful in all we do, which includes every run.*

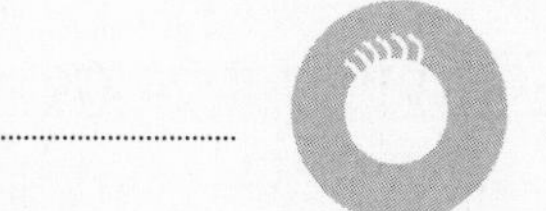

sticky notes

12
Week

the happiest race on earth

"Running God's Race"

THROUGH THIS MOTHER-DAUGHTER TRADITION, GOD TAUGHT me about togetherness.

So, what's all the hype about running the Disneyland Half Marathon, which now sells out in an hour, despite being the most expensive half marathon in the world? My favorite spectator poster on the course last year at Mile 10 said, "Keep going! Only $44.67 left!" And yet, I continued for the fifth year in a row to pay the exorbitant registration fee, travel, and hotel costs for this one "magical" race, but why do folks like me buy into all the hype? One word: tradition.

This race has now become a mother-daughter tradition. Why are traditions so important? Proverbs 3:1-4 comes to mind: "My son, do not forget my teaching, but keep my commands in your heart, for they will prolong your life many years and bring you peace and prosperity. Let love and faithfulness never leave you; bind them around your neck, write them on the tablet of your heart. Then you will win favor and a good name in the sight of God and man." Bind them around your neck-like a giant Disney medal? Okay, that might be a stretch, but one that helps me visualize a beautiful picture of what God deems worthy to pass on to our children. Life events, achievements, milestones, and circumstances - these will come and go. Some will be marked with grand celebrations, and some with flowers or a card. Most will be remembered in photos and some may be painfully forgotten. God knows our hearts. After all, He did create them. He knows we long for emotional ties, for deeper relationships, to be understood, and to create meaningful, lasting memories. The giant Disney medal reminds me of God's love and faithfulness, year after year.

A lot of life has happened since I first talked Natalie into running this race with me and a lot of life missed. I think about the many times I came home from work emotionally drained and too tired to make dinner, much less know the struggles of my kids. Too tired to listen to Dave talk about amazing new clients finally closing escrow on their dream home. Too preoccupied with students struggling in my own class, too many essays and worksheets to grade, and too many repetitive phone calls from my mom reminding me that her memory was starting to fail. It's not that the medal or going to Disneyland makes it all better or erases a year's worth of failures. Rather, it's one of many God-given opportunities to create new memories and to bond with my child. In the heart of Disneyland there stands the famous statue of Walt Disney holding Mickey's hand. Simply named "Partners," this statue represents Walt's vision when creating his magical theme park: "I think most of all what I want Disneyland to be is a happy place where parents and children can have fun together." Together, a word that has taken me nearly a lifetime to realize its importance.

I love that J.R.R. Tolkien wrote in The Fellowship of the Ring, "Books ought to have good endings. How would this do: and they all settled down and lived together happily ever after?" Most fairy tale endings omit the word "together." I suppose togetherness is implied, but what I have come to realize recently is that I need to be very intentional about togetherness. I need to plan it, carve out time for it, implement it, prioritize it, do it, and find joy in it.

When my husband and I were dating, a defining point in our relationship came when we found we could enjoy each other's company at a laundromat just folding laundry. Finding joy in the mundane. It really didn't matter what we were doing, the point was just being together. I have also found this point to be true in my relationship with Jesus. I have often sought out remote, scenic locations to spend time reading my Bible and chatting it up with God. I don't have to go very far; several parks in our neighborhood are nice, as is the nearby Lafayette Reservoir which also makes for a great hill run after my coffee and devotional time. Last Easter vacation, I was feeling restless and drove out to Monterey by myself for a run along the coast thinking that would bring me peace and "togetherness" with the Lord. It ended up being a really long drive, an average run, and not the awe-filled-heard-angels-singing experience I tried to manufacture that day. I was reminded that God just wants to be with little ole me every day, every moment, even in the most mundane activities and places. The cost for this lesson: a tank of gas. The benefits are priceless, and so was our fifth year running the Disneyland Half Marathon.

The race itself has never been a PR (personal record) type of event since many runners stop to pose with the many Disney characters along the route. Who can resist the photo opportunity running through the famed castle? Countless memories are now attached to these Disney icons with every turn on the course. Speaking of the course, it is not limited to the theme parks as it traverses its way to Angel Stadium via major streets of Anaheim. Once inside the stadium, Disney manages to assemble crowds of volunteer organizations such as Girl and Boy Scout troops (rewarded with free Disney admission for their 5 am appearance) to cheer runners on. It reminds me of Hebrews 12:1 “Therefore, since we are surrounded by such a great cloud of witnesses...” Met by applause, high fives, posters, and cheers, runners also catch their images on the jumbo-tron as the announcer calls out names electronically received from the timing chips on race bibs. Yes, it is kind of cool to hear “Irene from San Ramon” booming over the speakers in that special announcer voice. This year, a non-audible voice also cheered me on when I needed it most. I usually hate Mile 11 since the heat of the day has hit the streets, it is not a particularly interesting part of the route, and I’m just tired. I even prayed specifically this day for this section of the run to go by faster or to just run it with a better attitude. Almost right after the Mile 11 signage, a runner with a lime green t-shirt appeared in front of me. The back of his shirt had Isaiah 40:31 written: “But those who hope in the Lord will renew their strength. They will soar on wings like eagles; they will RUN and not grow weary, they will walk and not be faint.” Funny thing, the last two miles weren’t so bad after that. Together. A word that embodies so much of what running has come to mean in my life. I often receive the most clarity when I am running. Heightened prayers, verses illustrated before my eyes, coming to the end of my own abilities, and learning to run in Jesus’ footsteps. You could say that running alone has taught me the importance of running together.

Irene Tang – *San Ramon, CA*

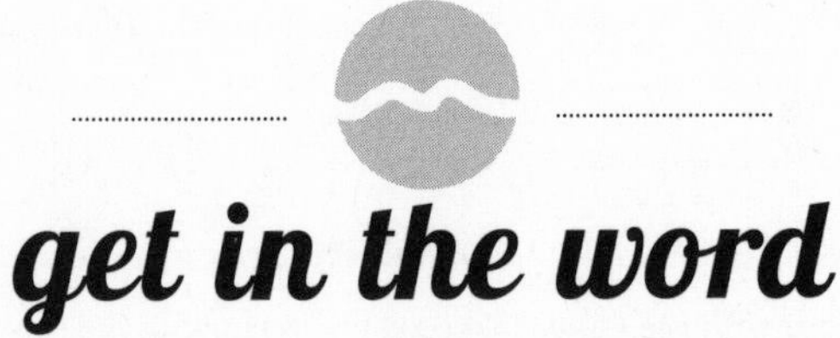

get in the word

Proverbs 3:1-4

My son, do not forget my law, but let your heart keep my commands; for length of days and long life and peace they will add to you. Let not mercy and truth forsake you; bind them around your neck, write them on the tablet of your heart, and so find favor and high esteem in the sight of God and man.

Isaiah 40:31

But those who wait on the Lord shall renew their strength; they shall mount up with wings like eagles, they shall run and not be weary, they shall walk and not faint.

Hebrews 12:1

Therefore we also, since we are surrounded by so great a cloud of witnesses, let us lay aside every weight, and the sin which so easily ensnares us, and let us run with endurance the race that is set before us,

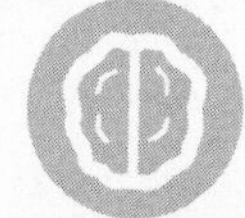

scripture memorization

Write out the scripture(s) in the space below and recite them ten times.

___

something to ponder

WHAT OR who does God use to cheer you on in daily life?

WHAT VISUAL aids help you remember key scripture?

HOW HAS God reminded you to depend on Him to finish the race?

running observations by dean

Accountability Partner

WE ALL KNOW ABOUT ACCOUNTABILITY PARTNERS and how valuable they can be. When I was in high school, I got up at 6:00 a.m. every day to run. That is tough on a sixteen year old kid! I had a friend that I would meet at a corner at one mile into the run. I didn't do it because I needed someone else to run with. I did it because I didn't want to be the guy who didn't show up! Accountability is a powerful thing.

When I talk to others about an accountability partner, they often tell me about their arrangement with their partner. What I have found is that there are different levels of accountability partners, from level one to level four. My accountability partner in high school was a level four partner, which I will explain at the end.

A level one accountability partner is one who you tell about your runs, whether you did them or not, how far you went, and indicate if that was what your plan called for. While it is great to have someone to talk to, who may even ask you about your run, there's really no accountability. If you don't run, maybe they encourage you to run tomorrow, but that encouragement may not be good enough when the alarm clock sounds early in the morning, and it is cold outside.

With a level two partner, probing questions will be asked that force you to tell why you didn't run. This adds a fresh layer of guilt to the feeling you already have for not running. It can be an effective motivator, particularly if your excuse is, "I just couldn't get out of bed." Verbalizing the indiscretion reminds me of the way I would feel when my mother knew I had done something wrong and she would make me say it, even though I knew that she knew. It made me feel a little worse about it, and I might think about it before doing the same thing later.

A level three accountability partner will ask about your run, ask for an explanation and then help you to find a way to resolve the barrier that kept you from running. Now you have the feeling that someone is in the boat with you, trying to help you row. When you have guilt, confess it, and then work on ways to fix the problem that caused it and you'll be making progress. It may be that your solution is that you are going to meet someone for every run, just as I did in my example. Not letting someone down is a great motivator and is effective in holding you accountable, but there is one more step.

I said that my accountability partner was a level four partner, and this is why: Not only did he know if I ran or not, he would ask me why. In addition, he had skin in the game by meeting me out on the road and providing a solution to the issue at hand, but he took it one step further. I knew if I didn't show up, he wasn't going to keep it between us. He was going to broadcast it to the rest of the team through good-natured ridicule. That was all the motivation I needed!

I believe God places people in our lives to hold us accountable for our actions. We know that the Bible tells us that we are all sinners, and many of us have particular sins that are most difficult for us to overcome. Sometimes, the only way we can change is to get someone else involved in our effort to rid ourselves of those actions. Proverbs 27:6 says, "Faithful are the wounds of a friend, But the kisses of an enemy are deceitful." We need friends and/or relatives who will knock us back in line when we need it. An honest, loving accountability partner can be just what we need to overcome a sin that haunts us every day. Satan is busy on the other side and he doesn't play fair. God has placed someone in our lives to help us overpower him.

- *Accountability partners are a great idea, but make sure they are really holding you accountable.*

- *A level four accountability partner is one who will provide consequences for your indiscretions.*

- *God wants us to overcome particularly difficult sins, and having a partner in the struggle with you can be just what you need.*

- *Are you helping someone be accountable to God?*

sticky notes

13
Week

to get lost is to learn the way - run your own race!

I THOUGHT I DID EVERYTHING RIGHT. It was my very first 5K run. I knew I was a slow runner and would probably finish last. I was at peace with that. Someone has to be last – why shouldn't it be me? I have never been athletic. I think it stems back to my childhood. Both of my older brothers were gifted athletes. It was not good enough to be average; I was expected by my classmates to be exceptional. My inability to live up to their expectations left me self-conscious and unmotivated. The fact that I could even entertain the idea of running a 5K was beyond my wildest expectation just a few short weeks ago. The day could not have been more glorious.

An unusual "Polar Vortex" had come down from the North, making the July temperatures unseasonably cool and more importantly, lacking humidity. The weather was perfect. I had all the right gear too - running shoes, special socks, running shorts, my runner's bib and my "Run for God" shirt. I was ready! I had been training for weeks. This was not a journey I had taken alone. Besides my Run for God team, my husband, Tom had been training with me. This was to be his first 5K too. He wanted us to cross the finish line together – even if it meant a slower time for him. We are a team both on and off the racecourse.

The signal to start the race was discharged and we set off. It didn't take long for me to fall behind the rest of the runners, but I was not worried – I had expected it. Shortly after the runners for the 5K began their race, a group of walkers/runners committed to a "1-miler" were released from the starting line, and I found myself mixed up in their company. These "runners" looked like the real thing, and like me, they had the right gear. They seemed to be heading toward the same destination; however, I soon realized that their race was different than mine. The course for the 5K was very specific. There were twists and turns requiring attention to detail. The 1-mile race followed a much easier course. I quickly became separated from my husband and the other runners in my group. Despite my best intentions, I ended up on the easier course to the finish line. I was devastated. After all my hard work, I had made a fatal error that cost me the personal victory of completing my first 5K. My team tried to comfort me, but I was inconsolable. All I could do was ask God, "Why?" "Do you not know that in a race all the runners run, but only one gets the prize? Run in such a way as to get the prize. Everyone who competes in the games goes into strict training. They do it to get a crown that will not last, but we do it to get a crown that will last forever. Therefore I do not run like someone running aimlessly; I do not fight like a boxer beating the air. No, I strike a blow to my body and make it my slave so that after I have preached to others, I myself will not be disqualified for the prize." (1 Corinthians 9:24 – 27)

At the time, I was not sure why God allowed this failure in my life, but my Christian experience told me that there were lessons to be learned. A few days later, a missionary friend sent me a bookmark made by a local African artist. On the bookmark was an African Proverb "To Get Lost, is to Learn the Way." I don't believe in coincidences. God wanted me to dwell on that thought. We all know that hindsight is 20/20 and looking back I realize that I was not fully prepared for my race that day. My intentions were right, but when it came down to it, I had not taken the personal responsibility necessary to properly finish. Because I expected to be last, I failed to learn the course that lay before me, and I became lost. I assumed that following my spouse and the others on my team would get me to the finish line. The hard part of this realization is that I was both right and wrong at the same time. I made it to the finish line, but I missed my race.

Just like our DNA is unique and distinctly our own, every Christian has a relationship with Christ that is the only one of its kind. It is personal, and there is no other quite like it. That is why in 1 Corinthians 12, Paul reminds us that there are many parts, but only one body. Every Christian does not have the same calling, but we are all working toward the same goal. All the participants in my race were aiming for the finish line, but not everyone was called to run the same race. I was following the wrong crowd and as a result I missed my race. Our Christian walk is much like this race. We set out with the right intentions, but our sin and immaturity get in the way. Sometimes, the activities that distract us from God's calling in our lives are not bad in and of themselves, and yet they can keep us from God's best for our life. When we fail to run our own race, we miss something special that God has for us. We can never have that back – it's gone, but by God's grace, we are not disqualified from winning the ultimate prize – Eternity in Heaven. We have assurance that our salvation is intact despite our failures (Romans 5:1-2). It is by faith that we are saved and, because of God's grace, we can get back on the correct track. That assurance gives me the confidence to move forward. The following Monday morning, I was up at 5:00 a.m. and running. There is another race coming up. I plan to be there, better prepared and giving God all the glory.

Pamela Emmett – *Glassboro, NJ*

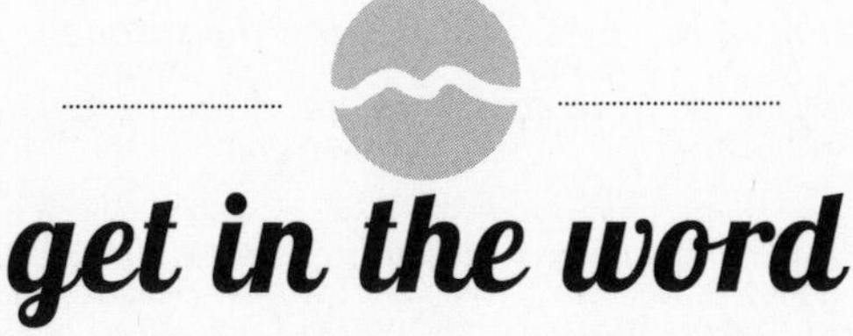

1 Corinthians 9:24-27

Do you not know that those who run in a race all run, but one receives the prize? Run in such a way that you may obtain it. And everyone who competes for the prize is temperate in all things. Now they do it to obtain a perishable crown, but we for an imperishable crown. Therefore I run thus: not with uncertainty. Thus I fight: not as one who beats the air. But I discipline my body and bring it into subjection, lest, when I have preached to others, I myself should become disqualified.

1 Corinthians 12

Now concerning spiritual gifts, brethren, I do not want you to be ignorant: You know that you were Gentiles, carried away to these dumb idols, however you were led. Therefore I make known to you that no one speaking by the Spirit of God calls Jesus accursed, and no one can say that Jesus is Lord except by the Holy Spirit.
There are diversities of gifts, but the same Spirit. There are differences of ministries, but the same Lord. And there are diversities of activities, but it is the same God who works all in all. But the manifestation of the Spirit is given to each one for the profit of all: for to one is given the word of wisdom through the Spirit, to another the word of knowledge through the same Spirit, to another faith by the same Spirit, to another gifts of healings by the same Spirit, to another the working of miracles, to another prophecy, to another discerning of spirits, to another different kinds of tongues, to another the interpretation of tongues. But one and the same Spirit works all these things, distributing to each one individually as He wills.

For as the body is one and has many members, but all the members of that one body, being many, are one body, so also is Christ. For by one Spirit we were all baptized into one body—whether Jews or Greeks, whether slaves or free—and have all been made to drink into one Spirit. For in fact the body is not one member but many.
If the foot should say, "Because I am not a hand, I am not of the body," is it therefore not of the body? And if the ear should say,

"Because I am not an eye, I am not of the body," is it therefore not of the body? If the whole body were an eye, where would be the hearing? If the whole were hearing, where would be the smelling? But now God has set the members, each one of them, in the body just as He pleased. And if they were all one member, where would the body be?

But now indeed there are many members, yet one body. And the eye cannot say to the hand, "I have no need of you"; nor again the head to the feet, "I have no need of you." No, much rather, those members of the body which seem to be weaker are necessary. And those members of the body which we think to be less honorable, on these we bestow greater honor; and our unpresentable parts have greater modesty, but our presentable parts have no need. But God composed the body, having given greater honor to that part which lacks it, that there should be no schism in the body, but that the members should have the same care for one another. And if one member suffers, all the members suffer with it; or if one member is honored, all the members rejoice with it.

Now you are the body of Christ, and members individually. And God has appointed these in the church: first apostles, second prophets, third teachers, after that miracles, then gifts of healings, helps, administrations, varieties of tongues. Are all apostles? Are all prophets? Are all teachers? Are all workers of miracles? Do all have gifts of healings? Do all speak with tongues? Do all interpret? But earnestly desire the best gifts. And yet I show you a more excellent way.

Romans 5:1-2
Therefore, having been justified by faith, we have peace with God through our Lord Jesus Christ, through whom also we have access by faith into this grace in which we stand, and rejoice in hope of the glory of God.

scripture memorization

Write out the scripture(s) in the space below and recite them ten times.

something to ponder

THINK OF a time when you planned and prepared for something that did not turn out the way you expected. Why was that, and what did God show you through that experience?

____

____

____

____

THINKING OF your Christian walk, what does it mean for you to Run Your Own Race?

____

____

____

____

HOW WILL you prepare? What is required of you to follow the course that God has set before you?

____

____

running observations by dean

Thoughts on Running Shoes

GOING TO THE LOCAL RUNNING STORE to buy some new kicks is exhilarating on one hand, but can be fraught with confusion, misinformation and anxiety on the other. If you know exactly what you want, a new pair of shoes is like a warm blanket on a cold day. But, if you're not certain, trying to find the right pair of running shoes is like choosing a new car. It's exciting, but it feels like a big commitment. You hope that they feel great after you take them home, but there's no way to know for sure that they will be the same after the test drive. Rely on the professional to guide you to the right choice.

I remember a time when there were only a handful of shoes to choose from. You would try them on and purchase whatever felt the best. Since there were only a dozen choices, it wasn't difficult once you eliminated half of them because they felt like bricks on your feet. Once you made your choice, it never crossed your mind that you didn't make the best choice. Henry Ford, after the adoption of the assembly line process, writes about color choice for his model T, "Any customer can have a car painted any color he wants so long as it is black." It wasn't quite the same with running shoes, but it seemed close.

Just like we find cars in every shape, size and color today, running shoe models are more plentiful than my childhood baseball card collection. There are more choices from a single manufacturer than there was from all manufacturers not too many years ago. It makes the shopping more exciting, but much more daunting as well. When you walk up to a wall of running shoes, it seems difficult just to find a starting point, but it doesn't have to be that way.

Once you realize that shoes not only look different, but they're made for different types of runners, you can narrow your choices substantially. This leads me to my point. I am often asked a question like, "What's the best running shoe?" I always tell them the same thing, "There is no one best shoe." There may be a best shoe for you, but that shoe is not necessarily good for someone else. Their foot strike and pronation tendencies could be completely different. I have heard, more times than I can remember, that one particular brand of shoe is the best. Once again, there is no one best shoe manufacturer. There are many excellent manufacturers out there and just because you wear one company's shoe today doesn't mean that it will be the best for you in the future.

My philosophy is simple, find a shoe that you like and stick with it. Don't change just because you want something different. Today, I am in my sixteenth consecutive pair of the same shoe. I found one I like. Of course, sometimes a company will discontinue making the same shoe and you will have to change, but resist changing until that happens. In my case, the shoe has been updated four times, but the shoe has remained largely unchanged. I won't change until they quit making it.

One other thing gets in the way of getting the right shoe for the right person. Some people are so fixated on the color and general look of a shoe that they pass over the shoe that would be best for them. Your body will appreciate you more if you forget about the look of the shoe and focus on the feel of the shoe. I realize this is an unpopular sentiment, but I have seen many runners in the wrong shoe because they liked the way it looked. Don't do that to yourself!

Finally, when you hear about the latest must-have technology in running shoes, proceed with caution. A few years back the running world was overwhelmed with the concept of minimalism. The premise is that a minimalist running shoe forces a person to run with proper form, landing mid-foot instead of on the heel. The traditional running shoe encourages heel striking because of the thick, soft heel. There have been many who have been transformed by minimal running shoes, but there have also been many injuries. These shoes are not meant for everyone. Likewise, there is a new trend in the other direction, making shoes that have more cushioning than ever. Again, there will be a large number of runners for whom these shoes will be the best they have ever worn, and that goes to prove my point. The minimal shoe and the over-cushioned shoe are on opposite ends of the spectrum. The fact that runners thrive in both tells me that it is important to find the best shoe for you!

God made us, as people, with much more diversity than running shoes. We are all on different paths, some slightly different from ours, some radically different. While there are an infinite number of personal routes we can travel through life, there is one path that must be the same for everyone: There is only one way to Heaven. Jesus said in John 14:6, "I am the way, the truth, and the life. No one comes to the Father except through Me." Although there are many people who believe there are multiple ways to heaven, he leaves no doubt. The only way we are saved is through a life transforming relationship with Jesus Christ. Don't be swayed by fancy marketing schemes when it comes to running shoes, but more importantly, look to the Bible to find answers to the most important questions of life.

- *There are many running shoe choices and finding the best one for you can be an adventure. To get the most from your adventure, go to a place where there are professionals who know about running shoes, like your local running store.*

- *Don't be fooled into buying anything less than what is best for you by looking at fancy features or colors.*

- *Jesus Christ is the only way.*

sticky notes

white line running

THERE WAS A TIME WHEN I ran/walked with only a destination in mind, and oftentimes, I'd finish really happy but feel achy and inflamed behind the knee. A trainer of mine assured me he could help and checked my form. I felt doomed to be plagued constantly with various health challenges and to spend hours in therapy with frustrating pain. One of the first things the trainer suggested to me was to run on a white line, so he could video my running form. I'd swerve, stagger and almost feel like I'd lose my balance at times. Sometimes my mind would wander and pull me to look in the distance and not focus on my path. His findings were spot on, so I trained faithfully and carefully on the white line as often as I could.

I had more energy, and my balance was getting better each time. I then began subconsciously running on an imaginary white line. Over a year later, having forgotten that awkward training period, I started meditating on the narrow way during a recent run/walk. I was actually a little sleepy, but I thanked God that I had stayed on His straight and narrow way, and I prayed for more of my loved ones to find it. I didn't even finish my prayer when I turned down the well-lit highway. The luminescent white line shone brightly in my eyes bringing a rush of joy to my heart. No longer sleepy, I smiled as my memory of my first white line running came flooding back to me. I eagerly sped down the white line with renewed energy. I thanked God that the white line protects runners and cyclists the same way that the straight and narrow way leads us to a sure run/walk with God. I ended with thanking God for more than a year of running happy and pain free. I urge you to observe and ponder your path...run on the straight and narrow white line, and you, too, will have a much happier and easier run/walk experience.

Wanda Harrison – *West Bay, FL*

get in the word

Proverbs 4:26-27

Ponder the path of your feet, and let all your ways be established. Do not turn to the right or the left; remove your foot from evil.

Matthew 7:14

Because narrow is the gate and difficult is the way which leads to life, and there are few who find it.

Hebrews 12:1-2

Therefore we also, since we are surrounded by so great a cloud of witnesses, let us lay aside every weight, and the sin which so easily ensnares us, and let us run with endurance the race that is set before us, looking unto Jesus, the author and finisher of our faith, who for the joy that was set before Him endured the cross, despising the shame, and has sat down at the right hand of the throne of God.

scripture memorization

Write out the scripture(s) in the space below and recite them ten times.

something to ponder

HAVE YOU ever found yourself swerving in your physical and spiritual run/walk?

Do you find it difficult to run/walk on the physical/spiritual straight and narrow white line?

HAVE YOU been able to thank God for how far He's brought you in your run/walk with Him physically and spiritually?

running observations by dean

Be an Overcomer

I REMEMBER GETTING SPIKED DURING A cross country race in high school and trying to decide whether or not to stop as I watched my white shoe turn red and brown over the ensuing three miles. On a steep decent in the first half mile of the race, I lost footing and slid into the runner ahead of me. It was a downpour and the mud on the course made it difficult to remain upright. But a good fighter doesn't stop until he's knocked out or the referee stops the fight. I had a good race and was happy that I didn't give up, even though my body was telling me to stop. The running world is rife with stories of overcoming obstacles. There are other times when those obstacles overcome us, and things go in a different direction. That leads us to a different kind of situation to overcome.

Gabrielle Anderson was an Olympic marathoner from Switzerland who took part in the first ever women's marathon to be run at the Olympics in Los Angeles in 1984. The heat of the LA summer took a toll on her during the race and she entered the stadium with obvious heat exhaustion as she staggered onto the track. Officials were quick to come to her aid, but she waved them off, determined to finish the historic race. The officials saw that she was still perspiring, which meant that she had not reached heat stroke level, and allowed her to continue around the track. It took the 2:33 marathoner nearly six minutes to complete that lap as she staggered and occasionally stopped and held her head in her hands. She finished that race in dramatic fashion to the cheers of the entire stadium. She was an overcomer.

At the 1996 Olympic Trials Marathon, Bob Kempainen made a move into the lead at 22 miles. With a 20 yard lead over his nearest rival, he became sick and began to vomit, but never broke his stride. Over the ensuing two miles he vomited several more times, but continued to press the pace and won the race. Although somewhat disgusting, it was an inspirational finish. Bob Kempianen was an overcomer.

Sometimes, adversity leaves a different kind of mark. The 1984 Olympic 3000 meter race was billed as a duel between Mary Decker-Slaney, world champion, and Zola Budd, running for Great Britain. Neither of these two great runners had spent much time running in a pack because they were usually so far out in front. But, this race was very competitive and they found themselves in a pack of four runners pulling away from the rest of the field. Just before the five minute mark of the race, Zola Budd went to the front of the pack. As she went around the curve she pulled over closer to the inside and made contact with Slaney. There was a break in stride and they became off balance, contact was made a second time and Slaney went down into the infield, injuring her hip and unable to continue. She had dreamed of winning an Olympic gold medal, but it was lost at that point. It left her with a different situation to overcome, the disappointment that comes from not being able to reach a goal. Sometimes we have no real choice but to become overcomers.

Overcoming obstacles are part of life. Sometimes we are able to hurdle them as they come towards us, like Bob Kempainen, and sometimes we have to climb a mountain to get there, like Mary Decker-Slaney. I often find myself working to overcome those more difficult mental obstacles while running. I think it works well, but it is only part of the journey. The real healing comes when I give it to God for Him to work out. It's a difficult thing for a competitor to let go of control and hand it over to Him. But when we do, it makes all the difference.

- *The running world is full of heroes who overcame great obstacles to do great things. If you're looking for another example, look up Billy Mills and read his story.*

- *As hard as it is for us to admit, there are times when we cannot immediately overcome adversity.*

- *When we learn to share it with God, we learn the meaning of Jesus' words when He said, "My yoke is easy and my burden is light."*

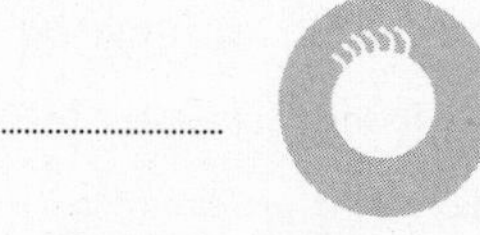

sticky notes

trophies of grace

RUNNING FOR GOD IS TEACHING ME a lot. As I ran this morning, I tripped on something lying in the path and it caused me to turn my ankle. I didn't think I could finish the run, but I walked and prayed. I was ready to run again by the time I got around the corner. I looked to see what tripped me and found that it was the head of a trophy. That next round I ran thinking of what had tripped me up in life. I remembered how The Lord had brought me through to victory in each one of them. I picked up that trophy head and ran with it this morning. I thought about how all my failures are as trophies of grace to share with the world. I thought about all the stumbling blocks trying to trip me up now and my heart says - No way- I'm RUNNING FOR GOD AND I AM GONNA WIN. I brought that trophy topper home with me to remind me!

Christy Hardy – *Northport, AL*

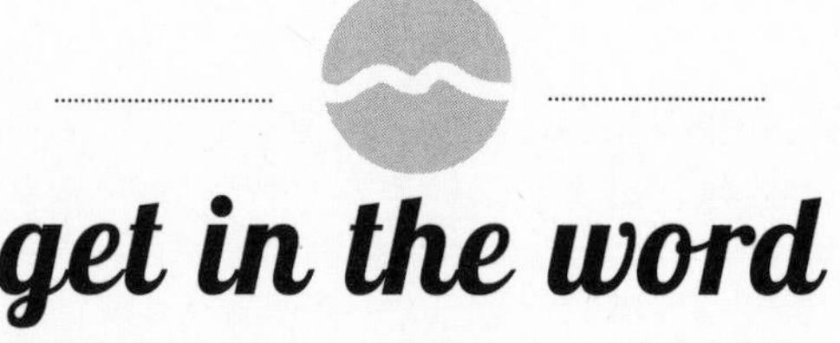

get in the word

1 Corinthians 9:24-26

Do you not know that those who run in a race all run, but one receives the prize? Run in such a way that you may obtain it. And everyone who competes for the prize is temperate in all things. Now they do it to obtain a perishable crown, but we for an imperishable crown. Therefore I run thus: not with uncertainty. Thus I fight: not as one who beats the air.

1 Peter 2:8
and "A stone of stumbling and a rock of offense." They stumble, being disobedient to the word, to which they also were appointed.

Philippians 3:14
I press toward the goal for the prize of the upward call of God in Christ Jesus.

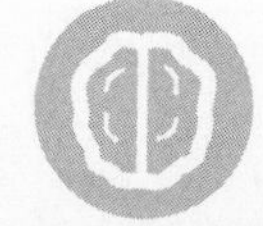

scripture memorization

Write out the scripture(s) in the space below and recite them ten times.

something to ponder

HOW ARE you training to reach your Heavenly goals?

WHAT HAS CAUSED YOU TO STUMBLE in life? How could you use those events as stepping stones to reach your world for Christ?

WHAT ARE SOME GOALS YOU NEED to press on toward in order to reach what God has called you to do?

running observations by dean

Etch A Sketch

THE ETCH A SKETCH IS A toy that began its journey to the National Toy Hall of Fame in 1960. It was invented by Andre Cassagnes of France and is still manufactured by The Ohio Art Company today. If you are one of the six people who don't know what an Etch A Sketch is, it is a drawing machine with two knobs on the front to control a stylus that displaces aluminum powder on the screen as you move the knobs, creating a drawing. The genius of the toy is that when you turn it upside down and shake it the drawing goes away leaving you with a clean slate. You can start over and create a better drawing, or you can draw something completely different. Just be aware, there is no "save" button!

Have you ever had one of those runs that you just wanted to forget about? Maybe you were sick, but forced yourself out the door, showing incredible will, but feeling terrible in the process. Or, perhaps you are still sore from a race or a particularly hard effort. Even worse, maybe it just came out of nowhere. You went out the door for a normal run and it turned south in a hurry. Whatever the case, it would be nice to be able to make it go away and start over, wouldn't it? Maybe not.

Those tough days are important days. You're not having a bad day for no reason. Even if you didn't see it coming, there's a reason for your struggle. It may be a stress issue, a nutrition problem, or an impending injury. Whatever the case, being able to run through those days will make you a tougher, more appreciative runner. I always like to say, "If you didn't have bad days, you wouldn't have anything to compare the good days to." Bad days are character builders, but more than that, they are opportunities to learn. When you have a bad day, don't just forget about it. It may be obvious why you are having a bad day, but it may be a complete mystery. Try to find the root of the problem by thinking about what you have done for the previous week. If you had a race the day before, there's no need to dig any further, but if the bad run came out of nowhere, think about what could have caused it. You may not be able to find the cause, but log it in your brain so that the next time you feel like that, you may be able to find the root cause in things you didn't know were triggering problems. Don't just turn the Etch A Sketch upside down and shake without taking a picture or, at least, forming a mental image of what the picture looked like.

There's good news on the spiritual side. Jesus provided us with an Etch A Sketch for our lives that we can choose to use if we have accepted Him as Lord of our lives. 1 John 1:7 says, "But if we walk in the light as He is in the light, we have fellowship with one another, and the blood of Jesus Christ His Son cleanses us from all sin." We don't have to live with our sins because they have been borne by Jesus Christ on our behalf. But the struggle doesn't end there. Just like we continue to have bad days no matter how much we run, we will struggle with our faith even when we have a relationship with Him. But unlike our running, He will erase those sins again and again. And, if we are His, we will try to draw a better picture the next time we place our hands on the knobs.

- *Unfortunately, we cannot just erase our bad running days like a picture on an Etch A Sketch, but they can be great mental strength builders.*

- *We should evaluate our bad days to find the root of the problem. Some problems can be avoided.*

- *God provided a way for our sins to be wiped away through His son Jesus. He's our spiritual Etch A Sketch. Like the toy, He doesn't place a "save" button on our lives. Once He changes our lives, all things become new.*

sticky notes

you're never too old

AT THE BEGINNING OF THE YEAR, my daughter informed me that she was considering participating in a 5k Color Run event in her hometown. She wanted her husband and children to participate as well. The idea intrigued me as I had not heard of a color run and it sounded exciting. Suddenly out of my mouth came the words, "May I join your team?" I exercise about 5 times a week in a minimal way, which includes about 30 minutes at a time just to keep my doctor happy. I am 60 years old! I've never done this before! Have I bitten off more than I can chew?

I began to ask God for endurance. Little did I know that I would be using His blessing to endure more than just the 5k ahead of me. I have now found I have strength and endurance for so much more, which I am using for His glory. My personal time with God, studying His word, has become the highlight of my day. He has blessed me with peace that comes from understanding His plan for my life. It is only with God's love and encouragement through His word that I can finish the race I start. I was the last one on our team to cross the finish line, but it felt great!

Kay Delano – *San Antonio, TX*

get in the word

Philippians 4:13

I can do all things through Christ who strengthens me.

Romans 5:3-4

And not only that, but we also glory in tribulations, knowing that tribulation produces perseverance; and perseverance, character; and character, hope.

James 1:12

Blessed is the man who endures temptation; for when he has been approved, he will receive the crown of life, which the Lord has promised to those who love Him.

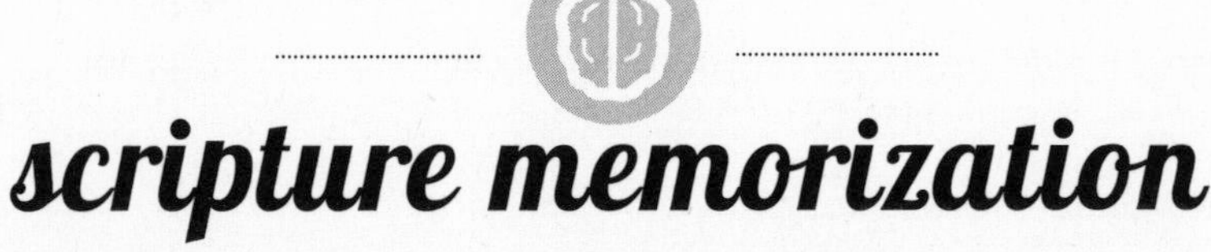

scripture memorization

Write out the scripture(s) in the space below and recite them ten times.

something to ponder

HOW FAR am I willing to go for God?

WHAT KEEPS me from achieving my goals?

WHO DO I know that needs to hear Godly words of encouragement?

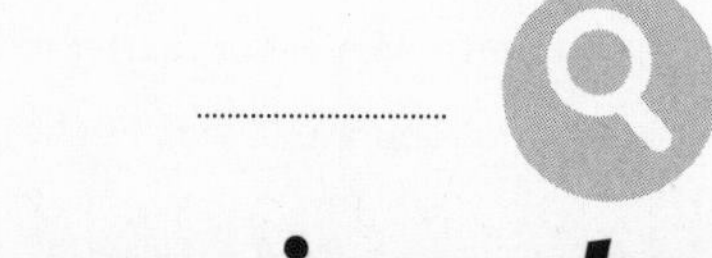

running observations by dean

Aging Gracefully

AS I CONTINUE TO AGE, I understand the meaning of Bette Davis' famous quote, "Getting old is not for sissies." As a runner, there are reasons to be discouraged about aging, but there are a surprising number of justifications to be positive, even excited, about growing older too.

Anyone over forty knows the aches and pains that begin to make daily visits, particularly in the mornings and during the first mile of your run. There are days, when I get out of bed in the morning, I understand why the average eighty year-old moves very slowly. If I had to feel like I do in the first five minutes of being perpendicular to the floor all the time, I would move much more slowly than I do. Likewise, as I try to get the muscles and other soft tissue loosened up at the beginning of a run, it feels like my joints are filled with molasses. If every step felt that way, I would be much slower. But, the body was designed for this. Aches and pains happen, but it does us no good to whine and complain about them. They're not going away. While we don't have to like it, dwelling on it will only make it feel worse. If you're whining about your age as an excuse to be slower than a younger person, they already know you're supposed to be slower than them. You don't have to make an excuse for their edification.

The other reason we hate to age as runners is how it affects race times. At some point, we are going to slow down and we are not going to like it. Knowing that you can never set another PR is discouraging, but it gives us the opportunity to wipe the slate clean and start from scratch. In addition, bad races are easier to handle because you have a built-in reason to run slower. Embrace it. Don't fight it.

Look on the bright side. The more we run and race, the more experience we gain, and experience leads to improvement. But, if we're getting slower, how do we improve? Running experience gives us patience, which is valuable for avoiding injury and making smarter choices when our plans don't go quite the way we intend. We learn how to listen to our bodies and make little adaptations in training that help to avoid injury or overtraining. We know what to pay attention to and what we can ignore. When we do have a nagging pain, we know how to address it because we've already been there. We let the young guys go out too fast in a race, knowing we have the ability to pull them back in later, because we're patient.

Runners have one day they look forward to every five years as we change from being among the oldest in our age group to being the youngest. It's a big celebration and is often cause to look for a race as close to the birthday as possible. I can't think of another activity that makes us so happy to get older, other than retirement. Focusing on a new set of competitors in your age group is a great motivator.

Maybe the best thing about getting older is the perspective you gain year by year. As you age, you realize what is important in life, and while running can be a big part of your life, it is not at the top. When you have a rough patch or a bad race, letting go becomes much easier. It's not that you don't care; it's that you have things in perspective.

The Bible portrays growing old as a normal, natural part of life. It presents the aging process as honorable, because growing old is normally accompanied by increased wisdom. Proverbs 16:31 says, "The silver-haired head is a crown of glory, If it is found in the way of righteousness." Gray hair was a symbol of wisdom in that time. Maybe the best thing about aging is that we have had the time to spend many more hours with the one and only true God, which allows us to be much closer to Him. It's no coincidence that the older people in church typically have closer relationships with Christ.

- *There are reasons to be discouraged about getting older, but there are also reasons to be excited about aging.*
- *The experience we gain as we make our way through different age group brackets helps to make us smarter and keep running in perspective.*
- *The hours we spend with God in prayer and Bible study have the cumulative effect of drawing us closer to Him.*

____

____

____

17 Week

the prize

THE CONDITIONS ARE NOT ALWAYS FAVORABLE, but in life some seasons are more difficult than others. The hills help me to remember that in every journey, there will be challenges. I remember to give Him praise when experiencing the relief of running down hills. There are times when others run along side me, times when I lead and times when I follow. I am mindful of when it's necessary to do either. I pay attention to what's in my path, so that I don't stumble along the way. I've learned that with every victory, I must become more disciplined, increasing the diligence and the determination to pursue the prize. It's not a medal, nor accolades from those who wish me well. Instead, it is the purpose. He is refining me. Running is just a means to an end. I know that my life encourages those around me and His light radiates from within. I am God's daughter and I enjoy pleasing my father.

Temeka Parker – *Bowie, MD*

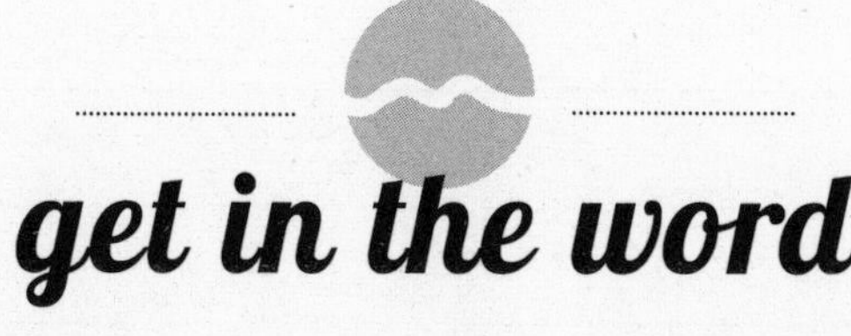

get in the word

1 Corinthians 9:24

Do you not know that those who run in a race all run, but one receives the prize? Run in such a way that you may obtain it.

scripture memorization

Write out the scripture(s) in the space below and recite them ten times.

something to ponder

WHAT LESSONS DID YOU LEARN DURING the most difficult seasons in your life?

HOW DID those seasons impact your relationship with God?

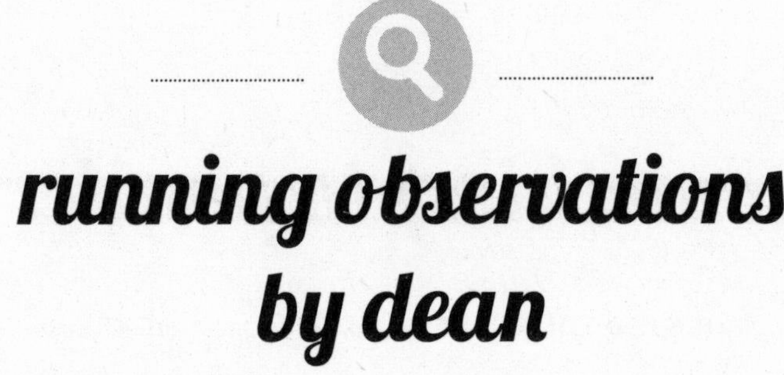

running observations by dean

Running Downhill

DON'T YOU JUST LOVE HILLS? CLOSE your eyes and think about a hill near you and picture yourself running on that hill. I'll pause.... Did you picture yourself running up the hill or down the hill? Most people think about running uphill. Why? Because that's the hard part, right? Well, it depends on what you mean by hard. While it is more difficult to run uphill, running downhill is actually much tougher on your body because it affects your muscles in a different way from every other type of training. As you run downhill, your muscles go through eccentric muscle contractions. It means that your muscles are under stress while they are lengthened, as opposed to the majority of our motions which puts muscles under stress when they are shorter.

The stress on your legs causes tears in the muscle fiber which leads to extreme soreness. It will make your ensuing runs tougher. I can verify the effect personally with two examples. The Boston Marathon is a net downhill course. You would think that, even though there are some significant uphills, it would be a fast course, but times do not indicate that. Why? The first four miles are all downhill, but if you are looking to bank some time by running those miles faster, you will pay for it later in the race. It may be easy to run faster in those miles, but the eccentric contractions will visit you on Heartbreak Hill because you have trashed your legs without even feeling it. The second example is a local race that I have run several times called the Chattanooga Chase. The first three miles of the 8K race are either flat or uphill. The fourth mile is entirely downhill, and the hill is fairly steep. It is always, by a very long way, my fastest mile of the race. It takes me three weeks to recover from this relatively short race entirely because of that fourth mile!

Here comes the good news, though. As you damage your muscles through these eccentric contractions, creating tears, your body will repair itself, and when it does, the muscles come back stronger than before. So, how do you make yourself better at downhill running?

Start slowly. Remember that the first session is going to cause a lot of soreness. You need to allow plenty of time for recovery. Subsequent runs will be easier and result in less soreness. Try a small grade to begin and work your way up to steeper grades. Be aware of your mechanics. Try not to over-stride. Although your stride will be longer than usual, the extra length should only be due to the length you gain from taking longer to reach the ground. Over-striding leads to landing too heavily on your heel, which will cause extra stress and more soreness. Focus on your effort instead of your pace. Begin by running on a two or three percent grade for a minute or two at a time at 5K effort. Wait until you feel your body has completely recovered before doing another downhill effort. Be careful on roads and trails, but especially on the trails. You don't have as much time to decide where to plant your foot. Roots and rocks combined with faster running can be a recipe for disaster, if you're not careful.

Paul writes in 1 Peter 5:10, "But may the God of all grace, who called us to His eternal glory by Christ Jesus, after you have suffered a while, perfect, establish, strengthen, and settle you." Sometimes life is tougher on us than others, and we have all had circumstances that were difficult to emerge from. But God promises that, if we rely on His mighty strength rather than our insufficient strength, He will carry us to the other side. We all know someone who went through tough times, and now they use those trying times to be stronger. Jesus told us that His burden was light and He would share the load with us. If we lean on Him in tough times, we will come out stronger on the other side. Like the pounding on your legs from downhill running can make you stronger if you train correctly, the stress from difficult circumstances can make you stronger, if you handle it God's way.

- *When we think of hills, we picture the uphill, but the downhill is much tougher on our bodies.*

- *If you practice running downhill, not only will you become better at running downhill, but you'll be stronger for level and uphill running, as well.*

- *God tells us that trials will come. If we handle them with His power, we can come out stronger on the other side.*

sticky notes

finding your sanctuary

I SPENT 40 YEARS WANDERING IN a wilderness. I found my relationship with the Lord while starting to run again. It was the very first time in my life that I spent quiet time with Him. I started running around a local city lake park. It was there that the Lord led me to fresh water and helped me to observe the fall and started giving direction for my life. It was in this season that I found myself without rest. He calmed my spirit and everyday I looked forward to running the lake and getting a word from Him. He directed me not to wear anything in my ear and said this is the path I want you to run.

He wants to talk to you. Have you ever had a close relationship with a friend? A friend you could talk to about anything and everything. I have had many friends, past and present, who have lent me their ears, and for this I am thankful. We go through seasons of change, sometimes good and sometimes bad.

Recently in my life, I have been able to let go of the things that have prevented me to hear the Lord through the Holy Spirit. I let go of pride and ego. Finally, I came to a time where I desperately needed peace. I couldn't stand the voices in my head, most being negative. I was going in so many directions, and I was talking way too much. I have always been an open book. Being too transparent, I have discovered now that it has gotten me in trouble many times. I see that there is a reason for my open heart and through transparency it can be helpful. Being transparent with myself and to my Lord has been the most beautiful experience and precious to me.

To actually quiet your spirit and come into the presence of the Lord in a technology aged society can be difficult; however, I believe, more than ever, that there is a time to become quiet. I encourage you to do several things if your life is in disorder right now. The first thing is found in John 10, verse 27:

"My sheep listen to my voice; I know them, and they follow me."

The first step is to find your sanctuary. Secondly, before you begin running, pray and usher in the Holy Spirit. Ask the Lord what He wants to reveal to you. Focus only on Him and His goodness. Stay the path and course that He gives you. Finally, when you're done with your run, you will want to journal or write a note to yourself. It is during your time spent studying His Word that He will confirm what He has shared with you during your run. It is in this quiet place that you will receive His direction.

Jesus said, "Come to me, all of you who are weary and carry heavy burdens, and I will give you rest." (Matthew 11:28)

When you can become quiet and let go of all the things that don't come from Him, He will start to strip those negative things from your life. He does this right before your eyes with the leaves in the fall. The leaves begin to lose their moisture from the rains that nourished the tree in the spring and summer. Then they dry up, wilt and fall to the ground. We are all infected and impure with sin. When we display our righteous deeds, they are nothing but filthy rags. Like autumn leaves, we wither and fall, and our sins sweep us away like the wind. (Isaiah 64:6) As winter manifests itself, we are in a season of cleansing our souls. When spring comes, the Lord will reveal all things fresh and new. This will be the time where everything blooms into blessings. It was when I went running that I found my special sanctuary, stopped striving in vain and became eager to serve my loving Lord. While running, nothing will compare to the time that you spend getting to know the love of the Father through His Son, Jesus Christ and the wonder-working power of the Holy Spirit.

Janet Carcia – *Chesapeake, VA*

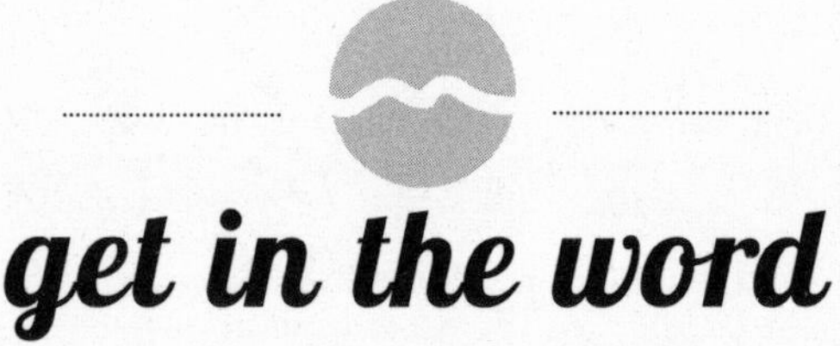

get in the word

Matthew 11:28

Come to Me, all you who labor and are heavy laden, and I will give you rest.

John 10:27

My sheep hear My voice, and I know them, and they follow Me.

Isaiah 64:6

But we are all like an unclean thing,
And all our righteousnesses are like filthy rags;
We all fade as a leaf,
And our iniquities, like the wind,
Have taken us away.

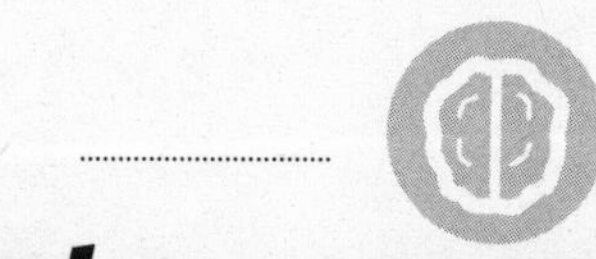

scripture memorization

Write out the scripture(s) in the space below and recite them ten times.

____

____

____

____

____

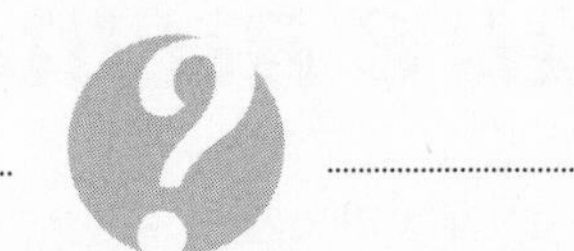

something to ponder

ARE YOU WANDERING IN A WILDERNESS and desire clear direction toward your promised land?

ARE YOU giving the Lord the quiet time and intimacy He desires from you?

HOW CAN you know the will, plan and direction for your life without seeking Him first?

running observations by dean

You Run a Lot More Than You Realize

Usually, when someone asks us how much we run, the answer is given in miles per day or miles per week. We are always ready to answer that question, but are we accurate in our response? I submit that we run a lot more than we think we do.

Trying to find time to run can be difficult with all of the demands on your schedule, so you often find yourself running out of time. Sometimes you find time, but you're tired and you don't run because you feel like you are running on empty. When you simply cannot find the time, it is because you are running around like a chicken with your head cut off or you are too busy running errands. With so much to accomplish, there are days when you feel like you're running in place, not progressing toward anything significant.

While you're running all over town, there are distractions. You run into people you know and when it happens often enough, you feel like you're running for office. Then you can't remember if you turned off the dishwasher when you went out, or left it running. After you decide that you did turn it off, you're off and running to the next appointment, but make sure you're running the speed limit or the police will run you down and write you a ticket for going too fast. You go into a store and have the cashier run your credit card through the machine when you make a purchase. Although not advisable, sometimes people will leave their car running while they run into the store quickly, in and out. They do it so that they can leave the air conditioner running, but have to be quick so that the car doesn't run hot.

When you're at work, you're determined not let others run all over you. After all, you can run circles around almost everyone you work with because you're a runner. You run to a meeting and offer ideas that need to be run up the flagpole. When your well runs dry and you run out of ideas, you run a meeting to brainstorm new ideas. Did you leave your e-mail up and running when you left the office?

You run home and run your eight year-old to his basketball game against the

Roadrunners. Any team with the word runner in the name must be good, and you discover they are as the person running the clock is getting tired because they're running up the score as you watch them run up and down the court. When you run back home, it's time to help him with his homework. You discover a lot has changed since the "See Spot run" days. You get your computer up and running so that you can run the computer program you need to get it done.

When preparing a nice salad for dinner, you run a food processor to chop up some walnuts you picked up from the store. With all of this running, you're going to need a good meal! As you eat dinner, you turn on the television. When you realize all that's on is re-runs, you change the channel only to discover that there is a run on the banks in another country, and hope that it doesn't affect our country. Sometimes we're so busy with life in our area of the globe, we forget the adage, "You don't miss the water till the well runs dry."

So, you see, you are doing more running than you think you are!

The Bible has a lot to say about what we do. 2 Thessalonians 3:11 Paul says, "For we hear that there are some who walk among you in a disorderly manner, not working at all, but are busybodies." Clearly, God wants us to be busy, but He wants us to be focused on the right things, not just running around performing tasks. In Luke 2:49 Jesus says, "Why did you seek Me? Did you not know that I must be about My Father's business?" Jesus is telling us that we need to focus on Him in all that we do. Sure we have to take care of all sorts of minutia, but we should be doing it with the intention of glorifying Him.

- *What's your answer when someone asks you how much you run?*
- *I always thought the word "awesome" was the most*

overused word in the English language, but maybe it's the hundreds of uses of the word "run."

- *God wants us to stay busy, but He wants us to be about His business.*

19
Week

being true to my spirit

I WASN'T ALWAYS A RUNNER, BUT over time I realized running was exactly what my spirit was meant to do. During a run along a long highway stretch where I was struggling with heat, I felt God's presence and my faith was rekindled. It took more time for that seed God planted to fully bloom. Part of the delay was myself. My doubts and worries, my juggling many aspects of life, my limited sight and understanding of the grandness God had for me. Today, I still can't see the full picture, but it is slowly coming into focus with dedicated Bible study, prayer, and truly trying to listen for God's guidance.

Fast forward from that run years ago to a recent race – the Maui Marathon less than a month ago. I had signed up for a running buddy through the I Run for Michael program – an amazing program that matches special needs kids and adults with runners. I was perfectly matched with Toby, and this was my first road race for him. His mom is an angel and prayed for me in my times of struggle and directed me to wonderful Bible verses to hold in my heart. On race day, I felt confident I would reach my big goal of breaking a 4-hour marathon, but as usual, I started falling apart around mile 16 at this race.

This race is my nemesis, and the second half was always agony, but this day things were different. Yes, I had big race goals. Yes, I saw them slipping away. Yes, record high temperatures were forcing me to walk. No, I wasn't upset. Yes, I said no more marathons. I said I wasn't going to Honolulu in December. I gave up on that, but not on running. All of a sudden times didn't matter. What mattered was my relationship with my husband, my daughter, and Toby. Those things mattered. At the end of the day a time on a clock meant nothing. I walked along the stretch of beach scenes I usually despised and saw God's glory. I was smiling and felt that this was perfect.

I recently read a book about walking with God through our lives, and I was walking with God. Nothing else mattered. I took the time to really savor the beauty in life and thanked the awesome souls who were out there baking in the sun to provide us with water, fruit, frozen flavored ice, and support. My eyes are tearing up right now as I remember all of the volunteers and police and how much they added to my day. But it wasn't all perfect. I lost count of the ambulances going back and forth --- more than ever for this course. This was my third time; I knew it was different. I said silent prayers and thanked God for providing me with the wisdom to let go of time goals and to finish safe and strong. I smiled more during that second half of the marathon than ever before. I truly cherished each moment and thanked God for providing me the ability to run every day and to run marathons.

My running streak started on December 30, 2011, so I know I have a lot for which to be thankful. I continue to run every single day. It is my blessing in life. I truly believe God wants me to run and to use running for a higher purpose – His purpose. Through running I have been able to motivate others to get out and start, beginning with my husband, but it goes beyond my family. I author a running blog to tell my story, share my hurdles, and tie into my gratitude to God. I have met many wonderful people who are like-minded and who have contributed to my spiritual growth. My running buddy furthered my reach. Toby has Down syndrome and was adopted from Bulgaria. Things are very different there, and I have learned so much from this eight year old boy and his family. Through running for him, I strive to raise awareness of Down syndrome; to make a difference; to advocate for inclusion of all of God's children – not just the ones who seem "perfect." Perfection only exists in God. On Earth we are struggling each and every day, and I strive to choose right and to lead a good example for my daughter to follow.

Ironically, it was Toby's mom who pointed me in the direction of Run for God, and I got instant chills. Yes, this sounds wonderful! This sounds like the perfect way to further tie my running, which I always say is my spiritual time with God, to my Bible study. I do not know what the future holds for me, but I do know this, I am strongly considering becoming a Run for God instructor in my local community. I have doubts. I wonder if there are enough runners on this small island of Maui who would want to do this with me. I question if this is the right thing for me. Is this where God is leading me? But I am not afraid. I am not alone. Through prayer and continued Bible study, I will find the answers. I will walk with God, and He will guide me to the path I am to follow.

Erica Gorman – *Kula, HI*

get in the word

Hebrews 12:1
Therefore we also, since we are surrounded by so great a cloud of witnesses, let us lay aside every weight, and the sin which so easily ensnares us, and let us run with endurance the race that is set before us,

Deuteronomy 31:6
Be strong and of good courage, do not fear nor be afraid of them; for the Lord your God, He is the One who goes with you. He will not leave you nor forsake you."

Psalm 32:8
I will instruct you and teach you in the way you should go; I will guide you with My eye.

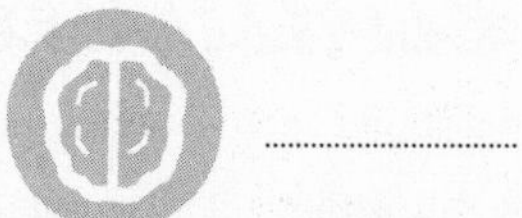

scripture memorization

Write out the scripture(s) in the space below and recite them ten times.

something to ponder

HOW DO you determine if you are following your personal wishes or God's plan?

HOW CAN the lessons in the Bible be applied to the struggles in running?

HAS TECHNOLOGY opened your heart to God's word? Please explain.

running observations

by dean

Open Letter to Discouragement

Dear Discouragement,

I only refer to you as "dear" because we have a long relationship. I have had you by my side so often that I don't even have to see you, I can feel your presence. However, you have been a terrible companion! You have lied to me, telling me I can't do things that I want to do. You placed doubt and fear in my mind and made me dismiss the idea of being successful in nearly everything I do. You have prevented me from accomplishing even the smallest of goals.

I'm tired of you! I don't want you around anymore. Although, I may feel you close by, I will no longer acknowledge your prodding ways. I will not allow you to talk me into lethargy and disappointment any longer. Oh, you can shout at me as loud as you wish, but I won't listen, and I certainly will not bow down to you as I have done in the past. I can't prevent you from visiting me and trying to persuade me as you have done in the past, but I will ignore you when you show up.

I have found a new friend to accompany me everywhere I go. His name is Jesus. He has promised me that I can get along better without you. He will never leave me or forsake me. I know you are strong, but He is far more powerful than you. As a matter of fact, he lives in me, and He is greater than anything in the world. I will be busy with Him and will become more courageous the longer I hang out with Him. I will be experiencing adventure as I have never done!

In addition, I will tell everyone what a big liar you have been! I will be sharing with them that I have found the Truth, and that He met me where you had taken me. He has set me free! There are many people you have inflicted with your lies and I think it's about time they know.

When you show up, I will meet you with a determination that you will not be able to overcome. I would tell you good luck with the rest of your life, but I wouldn't mean it. You will always be lurking in dark corners to prey on the unsuspecting, and even out in public places looking to smash goals and dreams, but I will be working against your plan for the rest of my life. Jesus has told me that I am a new creation, so my new path has already been charted.

Sincerely,
(Insert your name!)

- *Discouragement is always looking to tear you down, but you can choose not to take notice.*
- *The Bible tells us to "Fear not" 365 times, one for every day of the year.*
- *Jesus and His protection and guidance is the key to overcoming discouragement.*

20
Week

conviction

"COMMIT EVERYTHING YOU DO TO THE Lord. Trust Him and He will help you." (Psalm 37:5) Just two months ago, I was in the middle of a Jennifer Rothschild Bible study, Walking by Faith. In the introduction to the first week's homework, she asked a few questions, one being: Are you taking care of your body and health the way God expects you to? Now, you would not want to get me started on this fitness thing. My husband is in the Air Force and it's part of his job to work out, but me? I'm a stay-at-home mom and I get my exercise from walking the kids down to the park, pushing them through the grocery store, or chasing them around the house all day. Don't forget that I walk down the street to our mailbox every day, too. Isn't that enough exercise for me? I mean, let's get real here, I'm borderline underweight, so it's not like I need to work out. Even though I sometimes get out of breath making that short little trip to the mailbox, I wrestled with these thoughts and the conviction in my heart for a couple of weeks. "I don't even like to exercise." "When will I have time to exercise? I'm tired by the time Devin gets home from work. Do I have to get up early?" "Isn't it enough, God, that I read my Bible every day? Now you want me to exercise, too?"

It wasn't long before I couldn't fight the uneasiness in my spirit any longer. So, I found a Couch to 5k plan on Pinterest and decided I'd get up on Monday morning and go for a jog. I can only say one good thing about that morning. I did a lot of praying. I had to walk five minutes, jog two minutes, and then walk five minutes. That's all. I thought I was going to die, (Yes, I was really THAT out of shape!) but, although it was miserable, I got up again on Wednesday and jogged. It wasn't so bad that time. I made it through okay, and I was feeling pretty proud of myself, and then came Friday. I was supposed to increase my jog by one minute, and I couldn't do it. I made it 30 extra seconds and had to sit down before I passed out, threw up, or both. I felt so defeated and discouraged. I mean, I had pretty much chanted Philippians 4:13 throughout my entire jog. "I can do all things through Christ who strengthens me! I can do all things through Christ who strengthens me! I can do ALL ... well almost everything, but not this! Why isn't this working?"

As I walked home with my head down, I felt like just giving up. Who was I kidding? I hate jogging. I hate exercise in general. I'm not good at it, and I hate to do things when I'm no good. I decided God hadn't really convicted me about my health because He wouldn't convict me to do something I couldn't do, and it was obvious I could NOT run. I had myself pretty much convinced until I got into my Bible reading that afternoon and stumbled across Psalm 37:5. "Commit everything you do to the Lord. Trust Him and He will help you." Not some things, not most things, but EVERYTHING including exercise, especially if I knew I was being convicted about it.

Devin had been telling me that I needed to sign up for a 5k and it would motivate me to finish training. So out of curiosity, I researched local 5k's for the weekend I would finish my training. Guess what? There was a 5k in town and the day before that, a FREE 5k on base. I guess that was the Lord's way of telling me to, "get up and run." So, here I am at week 5 of my training and still moving along. I've progressed from 12 minutes of exercise at a time to 30 minutes walking/jogging 2 miles at least 3 times per week, but even more exciting than my progress in jogging, is the way my relationship with the Lord has grown.

Thirty minutes of walking/jogging at 5:45 a.m. gives me 30 minutes of personal time with the Lord. I have prayed prayers I never thought to pray before. I have poured my heart out as I watch the sunrise over the Santa Rosa Sound, and I'm in complete awe of God's marvelous creation. When I enter my one and a half to three minutes of jogging, I confess sins in my heart that I normally would push under the rug. The burn in my chest and the aches in my legs seem to go numb as I let go of things and give them to God. That bitterness in my heart, I take it to the Lord. Unforgiveness? I take it to Him, too. Selfishness? Jealousy? Insecurity? All of those things I don't even want to admit to myself? I take them to God. I commit EVERYTHING to You, and I TRUST that You will help me. Not just with jogging, but with everything in my life. Did God convict me to run so that I could better take care of my body? I think that was part of the reason. But most of all, I think the Lord convicted me to run so that I could run to HIM.

Danielle Wood – *Hurlburt Field, FL*

get in the word

Psalm 37:5
Commit your way to the Lord, trust also in Him, and He shall bring it to pass.

Philippians 4:13
I can do all things through Christ who strengthens me.

Hebrews 10:36
For you have need of endurance, so that after you have done the will of God, you may receive the promise:

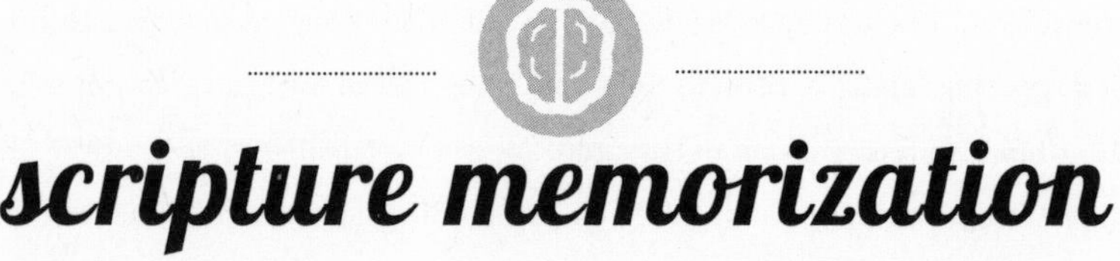

scripture memorization

Write out the scripture(s) in the space below and recite them ten times.

something to ponder

WHY DOES God convict us to do things we feel like we can't do?

HOW DOES running encourage quiet time with God?

HAS GOD ever given you Scripture right when you needed it?

running observations by dean

Wanna be Better at Your Job? Run!

A STUDY IN DECEMBER OF 2014 showed a link between the fitness level of the CEO of the company and the value of the company. A CEO was listed as fit if he/she had finished a marathon. The companies with fit CEOs reported higher profitability and higher value. The highest firm value was linked to those who were above the median age, above the median tenure and responsible for the highest workload. These leaders were able to be more effective at a higher age and higher workload because of the positive effects of physical fitness, including both physical and mental abilities. Not only did these CEOs have more energy, enabling them to get more done, but they weathered stress much better than their less-fit counterparts.

If you're a long time runner, these findings don't surprise you, because you have felt the positive effects of raising your fitness level. For example, being physically fit means you don't understand people who have trouble sleeping. Most runners sleep like they run, long and smooth. Of course, there are exceptions, but they are outliers. Many people tell me that they don't have time to run, but if you make time to run, you won't have to sleep as many hours to get the same rest. If you want the best night of sleep possible, get yourself into great shape!

A second tremendous benefit to the well-trained runner is the amount of energy she has. Part of the reason for the increased vigor is the result of the previously mentioned better sleep. In addition, a runner's body works more efficiently than a couch potato. Because of the training, your heart pumps more blood with every contraction, enabling the same blood flow with less work for your heart. Apply the same reasoning to all the other organs and systems in your body and you can see why a runner has more energy to burn throughout the day. I've been running my entire life, and I absorb constant ribbing about my inability to be still. My body doesn't ever want to stop!

A third impressive benefit to the robust runner is the increase in cognitive abilities.

Exercise increases concentration of norepinephrine which can alleviate the effects of stress on the brain. It also releases dopamine, which is the chemical released as a result of feeling pleasure. Any time we feel better, our brain works better, and we are better able to cope with anxiety issues. Cardiovascular exercise also creates new brain cells, improving brain function. The process is known as neurogenesis. In addition, aerobic exercise increases cells in the hippocampus, which is responsible for memory and the ability to learn. Runners are smart people!

With these benefits and many more, it is easy to see why runners make better workers. Similarly, a strong relationship with Jesus Christ helps in all areas of life. Although God promises us that we will face troubles, even persecution, He also promises to take away our fears and worries if we fully trust in Him. 1 Peter 5:8-10 says "Be sober, be vigilant; because your adversary the devil walks about like a roaring lion, seeking whom he may devour. 9 Resist him, steadfast in the faith, knowing that the same sufferings are experienced by your brotherhood in the world. 10 But may the God of all grace, who called us to His eternal glory by Christ Jesus, after you have suffered a while, perfect, establish, strengthen, and settle you." If we have a strong relationship with Christ, we get our reward in the end! Spending time in Bible study and prayer with Him is the recipe for a strong relationship with Christ.

- *Studies show that you will be better at your job if you are a runner.*

- *Attributes derived from running that lead to better work performance include better sleep, increased energy, and better cognitive ability.*

- *Strengthening our relationship with Jesus Christ through Bible study and prayer will help us in every area of life.*

- *Reference: CEO Fitness and Firm Value by Peter Limbach of the Karlsruhe Institute of Technology and Florian Sonnenburg of the University of Cologne - Centre for Financial Research.*

21
Week

i can't. God can. i'll let him.

ON AUGUST 28, 2012, I WAS involved in a near-fatal car accident. I was cut out of my car and and transported by Bayflite helicopter to a trauma center. I spent a couple of weeks at Blake Trauma Center and then was transported to a rehabilitation center for another few weeks. My injuries included an open book pelvic fracture, which is where my pelvis blew open like a book. The surgical team inserted a rod across the front of my pelvis with bolts on each side holding it together along with a larger bolt holding it all together in the back. I also suffered a broken tailbone, broken sacrum, crushed kneecap, fractured knee, broken nose, and a broken eye orbit. There was glass embedded in my body everywhere and my glasses cut into my face.

As a former half marathon runner, I was devastated when I was told I would never run again. I realized that I was wallowing in the dark and not giving praise and thanksgiving for all of the things that were positive in my life. I began to pray again and asked God regularly to guide me. In turn, my healing continues to be an amazing gift. I spoke to the first responders who cut me out of my car, and they told me they thought I would be paralyzed for the rest of my life due to my injuries. The doctors told me I would probably begin walking in March of 2013, but by December 2012, I was using a walker; by January 2013, I graduated to a cane, and by the end of January, I walked without any assistance. On 10/27/13, I ran/walked my first half marathon and completed 2 more in 2013. In 2014, I am completing 14 half marathons and have completed 7 so far. Without God's faithfulness in bringing physical and spiritual healing, I could not have accomplished so much.

Debi Lantzer – *North Port, FL*

get in the word

2 Corinthians 12:9

And He said to me, "My grace is sufficient for you, for My strength is made perfect in weakness." Therefore most gladly I will rather boast in my infirmities, that the power of Christ may rest upon me.

Proverbs 3:5-6

Trust in the Lord with all your heart, and lean not on your own understanding; In all your ways acknowledge Him, and He shall direct your paths.

Mark 11:24

Therefore I say to you, whatever things you ask when you pray, believe that you receive them, and you will have them.

scripture memorization

Write out the scripture(s) in the space below and recite them ten times.

something to ponder

DO WE turn to God when things are good, or do we only seek Him when we "need" Him?

DO WE ONLY GIVE GOD PRAISE for rescuing us from tragedy, or do we praise Him in the midst of trials?

DO WE BELIEVE THAT GOD DOES do miracles and that we could BE one of those miracles?

running observations by dean

Being Intentional

THERE ARE A LOT OF WAYS we define success, whether we are talking about running, what we do for a living, or what we do at home. Just like success can be defined as being a great mechanic or a leader of an entire division of a large company, successful running can be defined as getting in three runs a week and completing a 5K or running a marathon in under three hours. There are an infinite number of ways for us to get to that successful plateau or moment. Training plans and motivation techniques vary more than hair coloring choices in the hair care aisle. Not only are there a number of paths to choose, some are better for you than others, while another path may be better for someone else.

However, there is one thing that all successful people do. No matter what the endeavor may be, people who make a habit of being successful are "intentional." What do I mean by that? You have to plan to work and then work the plan. Being intentional means doing what it takes every day to reach your goals. It means doing it on purpose!

How do you know what to do every day to take you where you want to go? Let's think about it in terms of a map. I live in Georgia. If I decided to take a trip to Washington D.C., I would know right away that I need to drive north. But, I don't just hop in the car and point it north and begin driving! I will have to plan my trip. It may be as simple as plugging an address in a GPS device, but that device is setting a plan for me to travel. Now, all I have to do is put it on cruise control and head north, right? Of course it's not that simple. I will have to make the car go by pressing the accelerator, use my arms and hands to turn the steering wheel, and apply the brakes when approaching stop signs, traffic lights and slower traffic. If there is road construction, I may have to adjust my path a little. Although the GPS device gives me directions, it is up to me to carry out those instructions. Setting the destination, or goal, is the easy part. The ultimate success of my trip depends upon the actions I take along the way. When I am intentional about those actions, I will get there as efficiently as possible. If I choose to ignore the directions, I may get where I want to be, or I may end up in Wheeling, West Virginia! Each turn, acceleration and braking application is important, just as the food you eat, the rest you take and the runs you run take you towards your goal to be your best.

I am always amazed how many runners either do not know what their goals are, or they are hazy about them. But, if I ask the same runners if they want to be the best runner they can be, the answer is almost always affirmative. The problem is that they are, sadly, probably not going to get to their destination, because they are not being intentional.

Set your goals, plot your course, and execute your plan. You may have to improvise or take a detour, but you will know where your path is so that you can get back to it.

Do you believe God has a plan for your life? What are your spiritual goals? Do you have a plan? Have you spent time in prayer to ask God what His plan is for you? Jeremiah 29:11 reads, "For I know the thoughts that I think toward you, says the Lord, thoughts of peace and not of evil, to give you a future and a hope." He has a plan for all of us, and He will reveal it to us if we seek it with intentionality.

- *All successful people are intentional.*

- *In order to reach your running goals, you need to plan the work and then work the plan.*

- *God has a plan for all of us if we will seek it with intentionality.*

don't allow anything but you and God to 'run' your life

"SO, ARE YOU LIKE A REAL runner?" they would ask. "Umm... No, I'm just a crazy fast walker."

About a year and a half ago, I was propelled into a new season of life. As with any new season there were some uncomfortable changes that I had to endure that I would later recognize as incredible transformations within me. Several circumstances were out of my control and some of the variables were beginning to impact me personally in a way that I had never dreamt possible.

I am a very driven, goal-oriented individual with a lot of stamina and passion for life. I have a smile on my face and the joy of The Lord is my strength. I have always chosen to be optimistic and not allow "life" to deter me for too long. As does everyone, I have personal stories to tell about God's faithfulness throughout my life. Somehow this season was different, and it was a painful struggle to find hope, joy, and strength to carry out each new day. I no longer felt like the rock I had always been. I found myself in a real season of depression, the extreme opposite descriptor of who I was and who I am.

"So, how far can you run?" they would ask. "Well, I can run like a whole mile at a time and then I just jog or power walk in between," I answered. After several months of feeling completely deflated, I began taking even deeper breaths of God's beautiful life and love. I began collecting little morsels of hope. You know, "The substance of things hoped for but can't yet be seen" (Hebrews 11:1).

It is a personal priority for me to start my day out reading the Bible, praying, and journaling, but somehow I felt the need for more. I began increasing my devotion time each morning singing and crying out for God to refine me, redirect my course, restore my hope, and give me a new perspective on life. "So, you have really been running a lot," they would say. "It's a great stress reliever and time for reflection after a full day of teaching," I responded.

I began to emerge from this wilderness I had been trudging through, and along the path, I found incredible streams of living water. At each pool, I would stand in awe of God's goodness and reflect on not only where He had brought me, but even more so where He was taking me (Isaiah 43:19). "So how long have you been running?" they asked. "I did a walk/run half marathon back in 2010, but I've really only been running for less than a year," I answered. I had been looking for opportunities to network with other Christians, develop some new friendships, and challenge myself to do something new.

When I heard about Run for God I knew I wanted to sign up. Never having run a 5k, I assumed that's where I should begin; however, a few of my friends challenged me to step up to the plate and take on the 10k, and so I did. "Why do you run?" was the initial question of our first meeting. I have since thought about that question multiple times and my answer is that "I run for life. I run for hope. I run to give God all I've got for all He's given me. I run because it builds my faith." Running has become an instrument that buffs me both physically and spiritually (Psalm 31:24).

Depression is something I have observed in many others and have always found myself lacking in empathy. It is indeed very real and very painful. I believe 100% in a God who brings healing and freedom, and He is the primary antidote for all of our needs. Running has simply been an additional resource to living life to the fullest. I absolutely love life, and I am awake to the sunrise looking for ways to withdraw every ounce of life from each and every day.

Katrina Tinsley – *Cape Girardeau, MO*

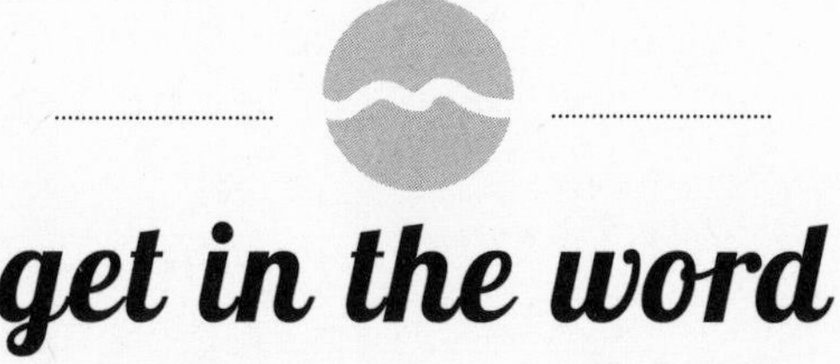

get in the word

Psalm 31:24

Be of good courage, And He shall strengthen your heart, all you who hope in the Lord.

Hebrews 11:1

Now faith is the substance of things hoped for, the evidence of things not seen.

Isaiah 43:19

Behold, I will do a new thing, now it shall spring forth; shall you not know it? I will even make a road in the wilderness and rivers in the desert.

scripture memorization

Write out the scripture(s) in the space below and recite them ten times.

something to ponder

WHAT ARE you allowing to run your life?

____

____

____

____

WHAT ARE some things that represent streams of living water for you?

____

____

____

____

HOW WILL you go about extracting every ounce of life of which God has blessed you today?

____

____

____

____

running observations by dean

If You're Not Enjoying Yourself, You're Not Doing It Right

IF YOU'RE NOT AWARE, RUNNING SHOULD be enjoyable. If you think any differently, you're going at it all wrong! For non-runners, or runners who think it is not full of joy, chances are that you focus on the negatives of the activity, but when you add everything up, the positives far outweigh the negatives.

Running is hard and sometimes it hurts, it takes time out of your day that you may be able to use for something else, and there is always someone better than you to make you feel inadequate. Those reasons are pretty substantial, but only if you look at them with an average person's eyes. But, you are not an average person. You are a runner. You are different! Sure, running is hard, but it makes the body hard and makes us physically stronger. Yes, it takes time out of your day, but being in better shape will help you sleep better and be more alive during those hours we are not running. And, of course, there is always someone out there who is faster than us. So what? Stop worrying about everyone else, take time to run "easy," and enjoy yourself!

After you take the negative properties of running and turn them on their heads, take a look at the positives! Is there anything like the freedom that running provides, or anything that makes us feel so alive? It's like being a child again! If you're the type to skip a run when it is raining, try going out to run in the rain, but do it with the mind of a child. Find a safe place to run and stomp in the puddles as you run through them! Enjoy the coolness of the rain. Be amazed by what God has given us in the form of rain!

How about having a discussion with yourself when you run? Do you have something to think about, or a problem to solve? There's no better time than when you're out for a run! It can also be good one-on-one time with God.

Remind yourself, while you pound the pavement, the trail or the treadmill, that you are making yourself healthier in many ways. Sometimes that is all the motivation you need to take the first step. You're losing weight, lowering blood pressure, building a strong body that is more resistant to sickness, as well as ensuring that you rest well. Whether or not you run for health, never discount the fact that runners, on average, have a better quality of life!

If those things fail, remember that running is not work. Really, it's not. If it feels like work, you're probably running too hard. Think of the run as half good rather than half bad!

Running is a little like marriage. It takes work and proper perspective, but the payoff is huge for those who do it right. Ephesians, Chapter 5, tells us that husbands are to love their wives as Christ loves the church. Think about that! It's a tall order, but when we follow God's word, our marriages flourish. If you keep running in proper perspective and take time to run easy, think positive thoughts and enjoy the experience, there's a big payoff.

- *If you're not enjoying running, try changing your thoughts from negative to positive.*

- *Remind yourself regularly why you run, especially on the days when it is tough.*
- *Like a God-filled marriage, running can be a great experience, if you do it right.*

23
Week

contemplating pain

WHILE GETTING BACK INTO THE SWING of running again, I was quickly reminded of the pain. I was listening to the song by Chris Tomlin, "Whom Shall I Fear." There's a verse in this song that says, "You crush the enemy underneath my feet." My greatest enemy at that moment was the pain I was feeling.

I thought about my own spiritual battles I've faced and how the pain of running are a lot alike. We start out with the first step into somewhere we've never been the moment of salvation, the moment when the transformation began. Like running, we are so eager to learn and to try this new thing that we know is going to be for our good. Then the pain comes through testing. Like running, you have to endure some pain for some time so that you can transform.

There comes a time when you've endured the pain, and everything you've learned starts coming back to you. You hold on to that feeling because you know your getting close to the finish line, and it's there that you gain a new sense of excitement - a second wind. You come to realize that the pain has made you stronger because of endurance. So, while contemplating the pain, remember that in the end it will all be worth it.

Errica Dana – *Crandall, GA*

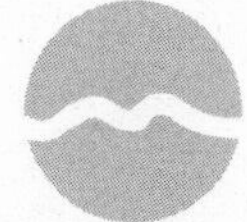

get in the word

Romans 16:20

And the God of peace will crush Satan under your feet shortly. The grace of our Lord Jesus Christ be with you. Amen.

2 Corinthians 5:17

Therefore, if anyone is in Christ, he is a new creation; old things have passed away; behold, all things have become new.

Hebrews 12:1-2

Therefore we also, since we are surrounded by so great a cloud of witnesses, let us lay aside every weight, and the sin which so easily ensnares us, and let us run with endurance the race that is set before us, looking unto Jesus, the author and finisher of our faith, who for the joy that was set before Him endured the cross, despising the shame, and has sat down at the right hand of the throne of God.

scripture memorization

Write out the scripture(s) in the space below and recite them ten times.

something to ponder

CAN YOU remember a painful time when God brought you through victoriously?

CAN YOU remember what great lessons you learned going through that time?

HOW DO you feel, right now, knowing you made it to the other side of that pain?

running observations by dean

Keeping Your Easy Runs Easy

CHANGING RUNNING SPEEDS WHEN YOU TRAIN is essential to improving fitness level and running faster race times. Most runners already know how important it is to run faster than race pace for short intervals in training, but some neglect the opposite end of the spectrum. It is just as important to run much slower than race pace in order to get faster. What? If you're like me, you fight this notion with your common sense filter. It just doesn't make sense, on the surface, why running slower could make you faster, but its true! Not only is there unlimited information on the topic, but I personally have experienced the benefits of slower running. I have tried many different approaches to running with over 50,000 miles of trial and error. I have tried hammering my body nearly every day by forcing the pace on my daily runs, and I have tried months of exclusively easy running (and a lot in between!). As a result, I have found exclusively easy running to be much more effective not only in making me faster, but also in preventing injury, as well.

Of course, the best formula is a mix of easy and hard running. Some can handle more hard-running than others, but a reasonable general guideline is to complete fifteen to twenty percent of your running mileage each week at a faster pace. Remember that there are no shortcuts. Trying to get stronger and faster takes time and doubling up on hard-running will only serve to slow down your progress, rather than hasten it. In addition, you will open yourself up to overuse injuries. Running easy will lessen the wear and tear on your body.

A great tool for controlling your running speed is using a GPS watch where you can see your pace in real time and avoid the temptation to run faster, or too hard. Be careful though, if you are not disciplined, knowing your pace could only serve to encourage you to pick up the pace rather than back down. I find it difficult to run slowly on days when I feel good, and wearing a GPS watch only encourages me to run harder. On my easy days, I turn the watch off and run by feel, keeping my pace and stride easy. I plan to run easy. When you go out to run each day, have a purpose to your run and stick to it. Often, that plan will be to run easy. A heart rate monitor is another tool you can use by keeping your heart rate in a lower zone and forcing yourself to slow down if it creeps too high.

You can also try running with a slower friend on easy days. It's okay to use them! Actually, depending how much slower your friend runs than you, the arrangement can be mutually beneficial. If her fast pace happens to be your slow pace, you can help her make it through her hard days!

Another thing that motivates us to sometimes run harder is the MP3 player. If you find yourself picking up the pace when you're listening to music, you may want to consider either leaving it at home or changing the type of music you listen to on easy days.

Finally, if you have a chance to go exploring while you run, the tendency is to run slower so we can see what's around us. Eventually, you'll explore everything close to home, but it's a great tool to use when you're away from home!

When I run easy, I have to remind myself that I am doing the right thing, even though it doesn't seem like it, because it's EASY! Sometimes, when I am reading my Bible, I have the same thought. When I have already read the same text before, it doesn't seem like I am doing myself any good, and that would be true if all I were doing was trying to check off a to-do item. But, when I keep myself focused on the real purpose, drawing closer to the ultimate author, I find new and insightful ways to look at the same Scripture. God wants His word to change our hearts, minds and lives. It says in 2 Timothy 3:16-17, "All Scripture is given by inspiration of God, and is profitable for doctrine, for reproof, for correction, for instruction in righteousness, that the man of God may be complete, thoroughly equipped for every good work." Reading those pages with purpose will make us spiritually stronger, just as running makes us physically stronger.

- *You have to spend time running slower in order to get faster!*

- *If you are one of those people who have a difficult time running slow, there are tools and tricks you can use to help you slow down.*

- *Sometimes it is difficult to keep ourselves focused on our purpose for Bible study. With His help, we can find both the discipline and focus!*

how Run for God changed me!

AUGUST 2013 WAS THE MONTH I made the choice to get serious about running. Before, I only ran to pass my Air Force physical fitness test. Even though I had six months to prepare, I ended up "cramming" runs the month before. There were several instances in the past several years where I failed the run portion of the test because I failed to prepare adequately. This time I decided to take a different approach. If I started running on a regular basis then passing my PT test shouldn't be an issue. Furthermore, I was going through one of the biggest trials of my life and I needed an escape to help me relieve the stress and pressures I was experiencing. This was when I discovered the Run For God 5K Challenge.

I first learned about the 5K challenge through a friend I ran with a couple days per week. At the time, I was already training with a Couch to 5k app and even ran several 5ks; however, I was very intrigued to see what this group had to offer, so I signed up for the Fall 5K challenge without hesitation. It was an interesting and emotional 12-week journey. My favorite part of the class was the Bible studies. I was truly amazed at how physical fitness tied into spiritual fitness and the numerous Bible verses that applied.

One thing I have come to learn through this class was to encourage and motivate my fellow runners. In the book of Hebrews, there is a scripture that says we are to edify one another. I remember when I first joined the class, I was in it for myself; however, as time passed, the Lord convicted me, and I started to change my attitude. I started to run with the slower runners and used the time to encourage, motivate, and get to know them. Before I knew it, we had our graduation race. Even though I set a new 5k personal record at the time, I had more satisfaction being at the finish line and cheering all the runners in because we are all winners. Why? Because they finished the race! After the 5k challenge concluded, I was ready for my next challenge- to complete my first half marathon. The first one I signed up for was the Chick-Fil-A Half Marathon in Athens. Shortly after I signed up for the Chick-Fil-A Half, I learned there was going to be a Run For God 10K/Half Marathon Challenge class with a graduation race on April 12, 2014, which was exactly one week after the Chick-Fil-A race. Since I enjoyed the 5k Challenge class and needed a training program, I signed up for the 10K/Half Marathon Challenge class in January.

During the registration process, I was pondering on what to do. My heart was with the Run For God group. My options were: cancel the Chick-Fil-A and run in the Run For God half, run in the Chick-Fil-A half and run in the Run For God 10K, and finally run in both half marathon races. My running friends encouraged me to run both halves, and the Lord reminded me that through His strength, I could do this. So, I signed up for the Run For God Half and put my trust in the Lord that I would not injure myself running two half marathon's a week apart. Twelve weeks later, I successfully completed the 10K/Half Marathon Challenge and was able to shave 4 minutes off my previous time of 2 hours and 9 minutes.

The roughest part of this journey was the Run For God Triathlon I completed in July 2014. After the 10K/Half Marathon challenge was finished, I was encouraged to participate in this year's Run For God Triathlon. At first, I hesitated because I am not a very good swimmer. Matter of fact, I haven't really swam since I took a basic swim class over 20 years ago. I decided to challenge myself again and signed up for the race. During the training, I was getting frustrated with the swimming. I got tired really easily and was scared to swim in the deep end because of my fear of drowning. Trying to schedule time to practice swimming was a challenge because of limited locations and hours of operation. It's easier to run or go on a bike ride. So discouraged, I was about to give up and quit, but the Lord used some of my friends to encourage me to press on and show me that I can do this. The Lord reminded me that He would be with me; I just needed to trust Him and believe.

Before I knew it, it was race day and I found myself waiting in line to start the swim portion of the triathlon. I jumped in, swam a little bit, and had a panic attack. A couple of the swimmers who passed me turned around to check up on me and encouraged me to keep going even if I had to walk and hold on to the rope. It seemed like a long time, but soon I did my 6 laps and got out of the pool. When I got out, it was like a giant weight had been lifted. With God's help, I overcame my fear of swimming. I continued on with where my strengths lie: biking and running. I was in awe of the amount of support I got while on the course, not only from my Run For God Warner Robins group, but also from complete strangers. 1:25:31 seconds after I jumped in the pool, I crossed the finish line and successfully completed my first triathlon. My goal was to finish it – I didn't care what my completion time was or if I was the last person to cross the finish line.

It has been an interesting year since I was introduced to Run For God. I really believe that, in addition to being more physically fit, I am also more spiritually fit. I can use my experiences to share with others and show them that through God, no matter what the race, you can be a winner. I started to wear my Run For God t-shirt at some of the other races and have had an opportunity to share my story and why I "Run For God." My encouragement to you is no matter what the situation, never give up, put your trust and faith in God, and rely on Him for strength. He will reward you at the finish line!

Brandan Keel – *Warner Robbins, GA*

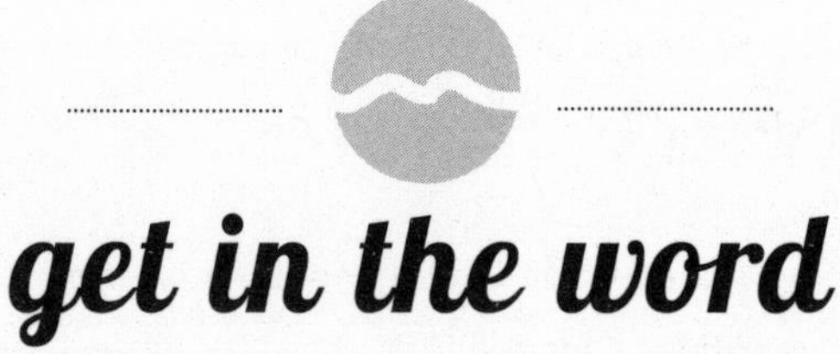

get in the word

Philippians 4:13

I can do all things through Christ who strengthens me.

Isaiah 43:2

When you pass through the waters, I will be with you; and through the rivers, they shall not overflow you. When you walk through the fire, you shall not be burned, nor shall the flame scorch you.

Hebrews 3:13

But exhort one another daily, while it is called "Today," lest any of you be hardened through the deceitfulness of sin.

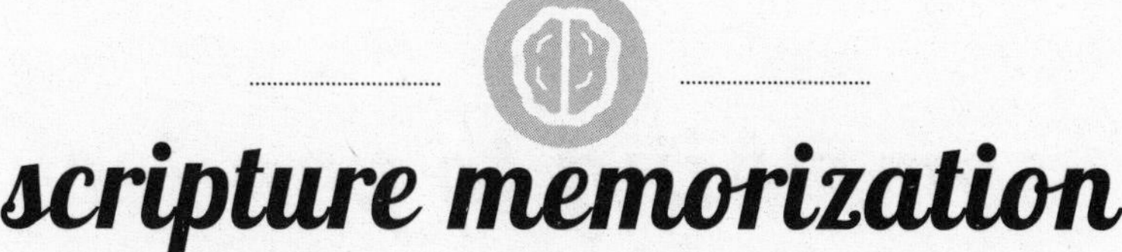

scripture memorization

Write out the scripture(s) in the space below and recite them ten times.

____

____

something to ponder

HOW DID you regain your focus during the time when you felt like giving up?

WHAT CAN you do if you see a fellow brother or sister discouraged?

HOW DID you feel when you completed your race?

running observations

by dean

The Enemy Within

INSIDE ALL OF US THERE IS a dependency on the known. We like the things we like and do the things we do because it's what we know. There is a force residing in our heads that regularly brings us back to a place where we are in control. It's what makes change so difficult for so many people. The reliance on consistency and routine is stronger for some than others. That's why we typically know people who are more adventurous than we are, but also some who almost never do anything outside of the routine.

One enemy that we battle is complacency. The idea of gathering enough energy to get out of the door to run is as much as we can handle. We convince ourselves that we're simply too tired to go for a run. We know we should, but we tell ourselves, "maybe we can make it up tomorrow after a good night's sleep." Overcoming complacency is easier than you think. Make up your mind, when the day begins, that you are going to follow through with your plans. When that voice tells you that you're too tired, focus on the feeling that you experience after the run.

A second enemy that haunts us is habit. We get into a repetitious cycle that can be difficult to break. I can't count the number of times I have made a wrong turn in my car because the habit has formed in my brain due the sheer number of times I have turned that direction. It's frustrating when it happens. The same thing happens to many who find it difficult to get into the routine of running because the old habits have been so firmly imprinted in our brains. Once again, schedule your run time into your day. Put it on your calendar and set up a reminder. Place a note on your mirror or in another prominent location until you imprint your new habit.

The last, and most difficult enemy to battle, is comfort. We're comfortable with our lives and the simple flow we have created. We know what's around every corner and what to expect in every situation because we don't venture outside our comfort zone. It leaves us apprehensive about things like going out in public to run because we're afraid people are looking at us funny, or to run on our own when we normally have a partner to run with. Maybe you're comfortable with running three days a week, but your friends are trying to talk you into training for a marathon. You know it will be difficult and will require more time. That's the enemy, comfort, trying to convince you that you can't do it. Don't let it win!

These enemies all have one thing in common; they are tools of the devil. Ephesians 6:12 reads, "For we do not wrestle against flesh and blood, but against principalities, against powers, against the rulers of the darkness of this age, against spiritual hosts of wickedness in the heavenly places." It's not us that we are fighting, but the one who doesn't want us to progress one step in a positive direction. The good news is that we serve a God who is more than we need to overcome. 2 Corinthians 4:8-9 reads, "We are hard-pressed on every side, yet not crushed; we are perplexed, but not in despair; persecuted, but not forsaken; struck down, but not destroyed." We cannot be overtaken if we have the power of God in us. The next time one of those enemies comes to your door to tell you that you can't do something, reach for the One who will conquer all!

- *There is an enemy inside all of us trying to keep us from growing.*

- *The most common enemies for runners to overcome are Complacency, Habit and Comfort.*

- *God is enough for us to overcome anything Satan can throw our way.*

sticky notes

inspiring without imposing

I JOINED A RUN FOR GOD group at my church, earlier this year, in order to train for my first 10k and to fellowship with other runners in our church. While signing up for the meetings was an easy decision, buying into the thesis of the curriculum took some time. Distance running is analogous to our spiritual walk? Is that what we're purporting? Come on! Maybe the Bible talks about running in a verse or two, but that doesn't mean someone needed to write an entire book about it.

If I was somewhat cynical about the connection between running and faith, our Run for God facilitator, Millicent, was not. She spoke passionately about how she had grown and changed over the years because of Christ in her heart and the sneakers on her feet. She felt the connection in earnest. Many Run for God participants featured on the videos felt it, too. It was real to them. In spite of my intellectual skepticism, I stuck with the training schedule and went through the motions at our weekly meetings.

I am happy to report that, somewhere around week five, God showed me the connection. I had gone into work one morning with gym bag in hand. (As a side note, I work in the physical therapy department of a hospital, so treadmills surround my office.) My coworkers noticed my bag and asked me how the running was going. I told them that the new shoes I bought, after a gait analysis at the running store, seemed to be helping with an issue I'd been having. I told them that my left foot was no longer going numb and that my time was improving. My coworker, Donna, said she was proud of me. She expressed an interest in running a 5k that our hospital planned to host in a few weeks. Another coworker, Kiko, said that he'd like to run, as well. During lunch, and when no patients were in the gym, the three of us got on the treadmills and ran together each running his own pace. It was fun, and the time flew by.

When I got home from work, my daughter Carrie talked to me about her friend who didn't believe that Jesus was the Son of God. At church, Carrie had been learning about sharing Christ and sharing her faith. She wanted to know how she could talk more to her friend about Jesus. This was, to date, the touchiest subject my daughter had ever broached with regard to her spirituality, and I wasn't sure, at first, how to respond. It was wonderful to hear that Carrie wanted to share Jesus with her friend, and of course proselytizing is part of our religion, but I wanted to teach my daughter to share Jesus with people in a sensitive, timely, natural fashion. I didn't want her to make her friend feel ashamed or embarrassed about her own religion, something that is important to her and to her family. Since they are only ten years old, I told Carrie that the best way she could share Jesus with her friend is to exhibit the attributes of Christ: to be loving and charitable, kind, forgiving, inclusive. The best thing she could do as a little girl is to be an example to her friend of how Christians' lives are made better because of their relationships with Jesus. Who knows? Her friend may make the decision to follow Jesus at some point because she saw, knew, and was friends with Christians whose lives were different, meaningful, because of their faith in Christ. I told her that if she were to be pushy, if she were to say, "What your family believes is wrong," or if she were to be rude or selfish, her friend may grow up to think that Christians are rude, selfish, and pushy.

I told Carrie about my experience with my coworkers that day. About running together. I didn't say to my work friends, "Y'all should run. It is good for you. Why don't you go jogging? Don't you care about your health?" That approach would have shamed or insulted, not inspired, them. My coworkers became interested in joining me on a run because they saw what a positive change it was making in me. They approached me, and not the other way around. "That is one way to share your faith," I told Carrie. "Live in such a way that your life is obviously made better by your relationship with Christ, and maybe people will get interested and ask to run along beside you." Carrie and I talked about Gandhi. I shared with her one of his quotes about Christianity: "I like your Christ. I do not like your Christians. Your Christians are so unlike your Christ." My daughter and I talked about what that quote meant. I told her to live the kind of life that would make Mahatma Gandhi want to convert to

Christianity. She told me that she couldn't convert Gandhi because he was already dead! She said, "This is taking long." I don't know if I made any sense to her, maybe she is too young for all of that, but it really helped me make the connection between running and faith sharing. And the timing, the fact that my coworkers asked to go running with me on the exact same day that my daughter wanted to learn more about how to share her faith with her friend, was perfect. God's timing is always perfect, even if my timing (final time: 72 minutes at the Run for God 10K) is not so perfect.

Ginger Anderson – *Calhoun, GA*

Luke 6:31

And just as you want men to do to you, you also do to them likewise.

Romans 14:1

Receive one who is weak in the faith, but not to disputes over doubtful things.

Proverbs 12:26

The righteous should choose his friends carefully, for the way of the wicked leads them astray.

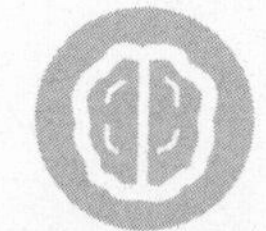

scripture memorization

Write out the scripture(s) in the space below and recite them ten times.

something to ponder

WHAT ARE some examples from scripture in which Christ, through His actions, inspires others to grow and change?

____

____

____

____

HAVE YOU ever made a positive change in your life because you were inspired by the actions and/or behaviors of someone close to you?

____

____

____

____

WHAT IS one attribute of Christ, which you would like more often to emulate, and how can you begin, through your actions, doing so right away?

____

____

____

running observations by dean

If You Think You're Not an Inspiration, Think Again

EVERY RUNNER IS AN INSPIRATION TO someone. That's a pretty strong statement, but one I can back up. If you will indulge me, let me share some of my inspirations. You will find that they come from places you expect, but also from some you may not expect.

I have been a fairly accomplished runner my whole life so I have an affinity for the really fast guys. I loved watching Mo Farah and Galen Rupp battle in the 2012 Olympic 10,000 meters, for example. I can't tell you how many times I have pulled up the video of Billy Mills winning the 1964 Olympic gold medal. Most recently, I remember vividly how I heard about Meb Keflezighi winning the Boston Marathon in 2014. I had just finished the race myself and a guy in a very tall chair was telling the finishing runners that Meb had won! I was happier about Meb winning than I was about my finish!

I help coach a youth Run for God triathlon team. They range in age from six to twenty, and they are a blessing in my life. As I watch them dig so deep for every ounce of energy they have in them, it is immensely inspirational to me. These kids could be doing anything, but they are pouring their heart and soul into the sport that I love so much. In addition, they are providing spiritual inspiration to those who see them as they run around town and around tracks proudly wearing their Run for God apparel.

I love going to middle school and high school cross country races and watching them compete. Running is usually an individual sport, but in cross country there is a team aspect that makes it thrilling to watch. Again, these young people could be doing anything, but they choose to give up their afternoons to run their guts out. I love it!

I run on a masters cross country team for the Chattanooga Track Club. The guys with whom I run, many older than I am, are an encouragement to keep going. My favorite race of the year is when we get together to run the USATF National Club Cross Country Championships. The competition among the guys on the team and other over-forty runners provides me with all the motivation I need to keep working hard.

Over the last few years, I have participated as a pacer for the Chickamauga Battlefield Marathon. The people running with my group are an incredible motivation to me. Knowing I played a part in a successful completion of a long time goal for these runners is something that will stick with me forever.

There is a lady named Gaye Coker who works with the Run for God team in customer service. She has no idea what an inspiration she is to people like me. Gaye is not a fast runner and is constantly joking about finishing last in races. She will spend twice as much time on the course as I will, but that is exactly what is so inspirational to me. Without her and others like her, races would not happen. She doesn't do it for awards or accolades. She does it because she enjoys it, and so do I.

Finally, my wife Debbie is a huge inspiration in my life. She is constantly encouraging me and looking out for my well-being. She knows I can be a loose cannon, doing things that are reckless and might expose me to injury, but she will gently persuade me to be more careful. More than that though, she simply makes me happy! She is everything that God intends her to be to me and that makes my daily runs more enjoyable. With the help of God, she has transformed me from an arrogant, selfish person into someone who has a heart for others. It was no small miracle!

It never may have crossed your mind, but you are likely an inspiration to someone. It may be other runners. It may the weight you have lost. It may be the way you treat others. Or, it may be your children, co-workers, or your spouse. People are watching you, and you are inspiring them!

My greatest inspiration comes from God. There is a popular verse that I have learned to lean on when I need a little encouragement. Jeremiah 29:11 reads, "For I know the thoughts that I think toward you, says the Lord, thoughts of peace and not of evil, to give you a future and a hope." He has plans for me! If I can learn to stay out of His way and follow His guidance, "I can do all things through Christ who strengthens me" (Philippians 4:13).

- *Inspiration can come from likely and unlikely places.*
- *There is much inspiration in watching other people run.*
- *God has plans for us, and He will be faithful to complete His work in us if we follow His will.*

sticky notes

26
Week

listening to my body

ON MY RUN FOR GOD THIS morning I continued to ignore my body's request to visit the ladies restroom. I wanted to finish "my run" first. Finally, it became urgent, and I raced toward home. How true that is of my Christian walk, as well. How many times do I ignore the Lord's gentle nudging to do this or say that, give this, and go there? How often do I want to finish what "I" have planned first? I want to go after my dreams first and foremost. Sometimes He has to force me to do what He wants me to do, because I ignore His gentle pleadings. He makes me desperately need to go, do, say, give, etc. He allows my health to fail so that I finally see my need to exercise and eat right. He allows me to stumble on things in my path to show me I need to focus on Him and follow His leadings to stay upright. He allows me to run alone to show me my need for a personal, intimate relationship with Him. He allows my family to suffer so that we might see how mighty He is when we surrender our very lives into the hands of The One who holds it all together. I want to quickly obey Him when I hear Him whisper my name. I want to respond as Isaiah when he said, "Here I am Lord, send me!" Isaiah 6:8.

Christy Hardy – *Northport, AL*

get in the word

Hebrews 3:15

While it is said:

"Today, if you will hear His voice, do not harden your hearts as in the rebellion."

Colossians 1:17

And He is before all things, and in Him all things consist.

Proverbs 19:21

There are many plans in a man's heart, nevertheless the Lord's counsel—that will stand.

scripture memorization

Write out the scripture(s) in the space below and recite them ten times.

something to ponder

HAVE YOU ever hardened your heart toward God? Did you have a hard time hearing Him since you disregarded His nudging for so long?

HOW DOES the Lord hold your world together for you?

____

HOW HAVE your plans failed so that the Lord's plans would prevail?

____

____

____

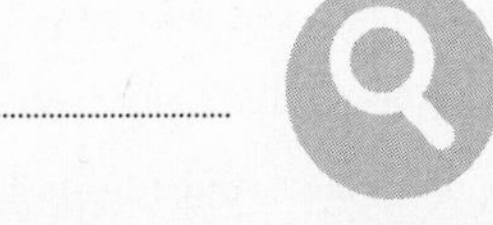

running observations by dean

Time Enough At Last

I LOVE WATCHING THE TWILIGHT ZONE episodes from the early 1960s. One of my favorite episodes is called "Time Enough At Last." It portrays a bookworm who takes every opportunity to read books, to the detriment of his relationships with his wife and boss. He would rather read a poem than spend time with his wife. As a bank teller, he tries to read novels while waiting on customers, which causes his boss to threaten to fire him for not doing his job. He is completely hung up on reading!

One day, he decides to go to the bank vault during his break time so that he can read on his lunch hour, undisturbed. While he is in the vault, The Bomb is dropped. When he wakes up, he realizes that everyone else is gone and he is the last man on Earth. He walks through the rubble and eventually decides to end his life when he realizes how lonely he is. Just as he is about to pull the trigger of a gun aimed at his head, he sees a sign for a library!

He gathers up the books and organizes them to keep him actively reading for the coming years. Then, he notices something on the ground, and he bends over to see what it is. His glasses fall off his face and shatter as they hit the ground. He picks them up, realizing he cannot see well enough to read and there is no one left to repair them, he laments that, "There was time. Time enough at last."

Sometimes it's difficult to find the time to run, but if we're waiting for some big event, like finding out we inherited a million dollars, it's probably not going to happen. When someone tells me they don't have time to run, I will tell them that it's okay to say you don't have time to run, but don't confuse the amount of time you have with your priorities. Every day still has twenty-four hours. When you say you don't have time, it simply means that you are saying that everything else you are doing is more important. And, if that is truly the case, then you will have difficulty finding time to run. However, upon further investigation, most will admit to spending time regularly on non-essential activities like watching television programs.

All I'm saying, trying not to be too meddlesome, is that if you are throwing the "I don't have time" card, make sure everything else you are doing is more important. Otherwise, like a friend of mine likes to say, "Suck it up, buttercup," and get yourself out the door to run!

The same excuse is the number one reason why people fail to find time for Bible reading. It's not just the lack of time that keeps us from doing what we know is best for us, it's all the competing things that demand our time. So what is the solution? Maybe a fresh evaluation of our activities would reveal that we are spending time doing things that we don't need to do. We would never go a week without eating, but Jesus said in Matthew 4:4, "It is written, 'Man shall not live by bread alone, but by every word that proceeds from the mouth of God.'" Jesus was saying that reading your Bible is as important as eating. Is there anything more significant than hearing from Him?

- *The difficulty of finding time to do the things we enjoy goes beyond The Twilight Zone episode from 1960.*
- *When we say we don't have time for something, we're really saying that other things are more important.*
- *Jesus tell us that we need the Word of God as much as we need the food on our table.*

____

____

____

____

____

____

____

____

____

____

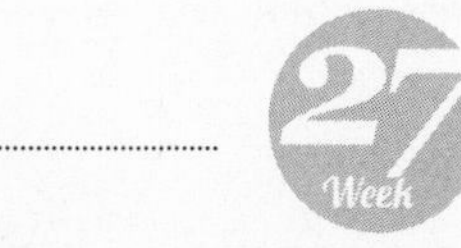

the great wall

WITH THE GREAT WALL'S MAIN SECTIONS totaling over 13,000 miles and earliest sections built 700 years B.C., the Great Wall Marathon is hardly a walk in the park. This marathon challenges runners to steep ascents and descents along with 5,164 stone steps. Whoa, wait, no, I most certainly have not run the Great Wall Marathon; however, it did cross my mind two years ago when our family was planning its first visit to China. Yes, scheduling races and runs as part of vacation itineraries is normal for us runners. Runner's World Magazine lists this habit as one of the ways you know you're a runner. As we stood in the long line waiting for the gondola to take us up to the Great Wall, I soon realized how uneducated I was about its significance. For one, I didn't know The Great Wall could be seen from the Moon. I didn't know the section of wall we were visiting was the first section open to the public, as well as the most frequently renovated and strongest as it once protected nearby Beijing from invasions. On this day, the seventeen-member Tang Dynasty invaded the Great Wall, along with more tourists than I have ever rubbed sweaty arms and legs. It was more crowded than the start line of the L.A. and S.F. Marathons combined. My dream of running on the Great Wall quickly faded as I saw that this whole section of wall (26 feet high and 16 feet wide at its widest) was more wall-to-wall tourists than brick - The Great Wall of Tourists. Annoyed also by the noonday humidity, I was determined to make my way through the crowds to find a cooler, less-populated section to redeem part of my dream. I did find some redemption as I ventured farther down the wall than most tourists were willing to go, since the trek down meant a steep trek back up. After escaping the most crowded sections, I found it quite pleasant and even relaxing to gaze out into the distance and see nothing but miles of wall and green mountains. It was surreal. I realized that to truly appreciate the greatness of this wall, I had to look past where I was standing.

In running, "the great wall" is really not great from any vantage point. Often referred to as "hitting the wall" or "bonking," I have fallen victim to visiting this wall many times. I've read dozens of articles to try to gain a better understanding of how it is I continue to hit this wall despite hours of training and proper nutrition. This excerpt from Competitor Magazine's October 2013 issue seems to cover it simply enough:

The prevailing belief has been that the wall occurs when a runner depletes his or her very limited reserves of glycogen, a carbohydrate-based fuel source for muscle contractions. The body stores plenty of glycogen to get through shorter races, but not always enough to deliver runners to the finish line of a marathon, especially if their pace is too aggressive.

That is the story of my running life.

How many times have I crossed the finish line and looked down at my watch only to be disappointed that I didn't hit my goal? More often than not. The obvious solution is to stop going out faster than my goal pace, right? Sure, in those first few marathons, I could blame adrenaline and inexperience. You would think that the physical and psychological pain encountered at mile 20 would be enough to ensure that I never make that mistake again, yet something happens after the starting horn goes off. I feel good. I have this internal dialogue with myself convincing me that I can somehow hold this pace despite training at a slower pace. I'm thinking personal record. I'm thinking, "Today is the day!" I even repeat favorite Bible verses over and over, such as

1 Corinthians 9:24, "Run to win," Hebrews 12:3, "I will not grow weary or lose heart!" and, of course, Philippians 4:13, "I can do all things through Christ who strengthens me." Somehow, when Paul wrote that verse to the church in Philippi, I don't think he was envisioning this middle-aged mom trying to run a sub-4 hour marathon. It is easy to take certain Bible verses out of context. Over the years, I have come to appreciate any verses that refer to running – and there are many, but that widely-quoted verse from Philippians 4 was actually part of a thank you letter written by Paul as a missionary dependent on the donations from those supporting his calling to deliver the Gospel to the unreached. Some of the letter in Chapter 4 reads:

...I have learned to be content whatever the circumstances. I know what it is to be in need, and I know what it is to have plenty. I have learned the secret of being content in any and every situation, whether well fed or hungry, whether living in plenty or in want. I can do all this through him who gives me strength.

Based on verse 13 alone, more people should be running marathons and qualifying for Boston, but as I look at my own track record, this mindset, ironically, has kept me from more success. I believe the key reason I have failed to maintain a more consistent race pace (leading to hitting the wall) is not being content or convinced that God's timing is best for me. Before any race – of any distance – I always ask God to be my coach, running partner, and pacer. I ask Jesus to "guide my stride" and "pace my race." Too often, after the starting horn sounds, I take matters into my own hands – and feet. I can't be content with my Coach's plan when everyone else is racing ahead of me. All of a sudden, I have selectively chosen to ignore verses 11 and 12 because "I can do ALL THIS through Him who gives me strength" just sounds so much better and easier to believe. Now, this in no way implies that God doesn't want us to aim high and rely on Him to do the seemingly impossible, but Philippians 4:13 can be a recipe for marathon disaster when taken out of context. It is a difference in perspective. Process versus outcome. Am I willing to trust that God knows the most beneficial pace for me to achieve certain goals in a race or in life?

We've all hit walls in life. How we come out on the other side largely depends on our perspective. Did I learn from my mistakes? Do I see this setback as a stepping-stone to the next great improvement? Is this circumstance exposing a weakness I need to address? Do I need to set more realistic goals by factoring in the cost to family and friends? Am I content with how God provides each step of the way? Sure, there are things I could have done to prevent myself from hitting those walls. Much like the way we should look at the Great Wall of China, we can't just look at one section to appreciate its greatness, we need to look at the whole.

Irene Tang – *San Ramon, CA*

get in the word

1 Corinthians 9:24

Do you not know that those who run in a race all run, but one receives the prize? Run in such a way that you may obtain it.

Hebrews 12:3

For consider Him who endured such hostility from sinners against Himself, lest you become weary and discouraged in your souls.

Philippians 4:13

I can do all things through Christ who strengthens me.

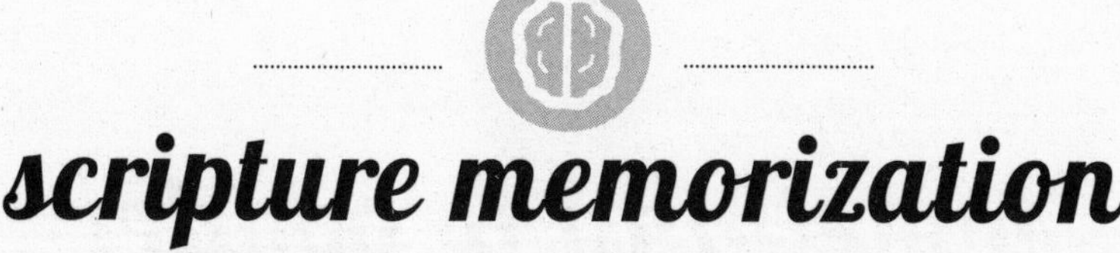

scripture memorization

Write out the scripture(s) in the space below and recite them ten times.

something to ponder

WHAT DOES "run to win" mean to you?

WHAT DOES it mean to be content in all circumstances?

____

HOW DO you rely on God to pace your race?

____

____

____

____

running observations by dean

Always in Control

ONE OF MY FAVORITE THINGS I do all year is run as a pacer in the Chickamauga Battlefield Marathon. Like many things we enjoy doing, I can recall so many great memories, from the guy who shared his story of how he had lost 80 pounds in the past year and was now running a marathon, to the two guys I have helped pace to PRs who broke their previous records by more than twenty minutes, nearly qualifying for Boston! But, there are challenges in almost everything we do, and I remember one year when I was in a panic before the race began.

As a pacer, the job is much easier today than it was twenty years ago before the proliferation of GPS watches. On this particular morning, I had a malfunctioning

GPS watch. I had thought ahead and made sure it was fully charged and I had a pace band so that I would know each mile how close I was running to goal pace. The pace band is also really important just in case the GPS part of the watch does not work. On this particularly cold morning, the button on my watch was sticking. I could not get it to change to the correct setting to enable me to time the race, either with the GPS or the stopwatch. I had not been using my watch for the two weeks prior because I was recovering from an Ironman distance triathlon and did not want to push myself, so I would not time my runs. Now, it would not start! Ugh!

With less than 5 minutes until start time, I kept beating on my watch, pressing the button over and over again, trying to get it to work. Oh no, I still had not taken off my warm up pants and jacket! Stripping down, I tried to think of a quick solution. I asked my wife, Debbie, for her watch. She was there to be a photographer so it was not as important to her as it was to me. She gave me her watch and I placed it next to my GPS watch, hoping it would not be needed. My next move must have looked really funny as I began to blow on my watch assuming the cold was causing it to stick. Finally, I got it to begin looking for a signal, but the cannon was about to sound signifying the start of the race. I ran to the starting line, looked around to find those who looked like they had lost something, and introduced myself to those who were looking for my pace group. I was trying to keep my cool, but I don't think I was doing a very good job. I felt like Barney Fife, trying to look like I knew what I was doing but looking really awkward in the attempt!

Just before the cannon went off, my watch found the GPS signal! Score! When the cannon sounded, I pressed the start button on my watch and looked to verify that it had started. Oh no, it was stuck again! I waited a long four seconds or so before I heard the familiar beep that indicated that it began recording. Whoa, that was close! It would be no big deal for me to adjust for those four seconds out on the course, and I settled in to my duties as the pacer for the 3:15 pace group. From that point, it was a great day and everything went off without a hitch, until about seventeen miles when my watch wigged out (technical term) and the average pace dropped ten seconds in a minute! This meant I could no longer count on my watch for anything more than a stopwatch. It wasn't the end of the world, but it would make my job a little tougher. But over the ensuing couple of miles, I felt God telling me to calm down. I thought, "Wow! I'm terribly concerned about such a minor thing, and He was in control the entire time." Over the last six miles, I left my worry behind me and just kept going, checking my progress at each mile, and it was fine.

I had short-changed God. I had not called on Him. He waited for me to let Him help me, and I had ignored Him for twenty miles. If you're like me, I'm always trying to convince myself that I'm in control. All the while, He is calling to us to let Him have control. When we do, it is so much more peaceful. He tells us in Matthew 11:30, "For My yoke is easy and My burden is light." It is so difficult, as we get caught up in life, to let Him have control, but He assures us that when we do, He will help us bear the burden. Once I let go during my pacing duties, I finished closer to my goal than I had ever done before!

- *Technology is great, but always have a backup plan!*

- *The joy of helping someone reach their running goals is even greater than reaching my own goals! If you have never had an opportunity to "help" someone through a race, search it out. You won't be sorry!*

- *God is in control, but only if we don't get in the way. We have to hand the reigns to Him to receive the greatest blessings.*

sticky notes

the sculptor

IT MIGHT BE A LOST ART, but my dad was a whittler. He was born in a generation where all boys carried pocketknives to school and regularly played mumblety-peg. I was never taught the game that featured sticking a knife in the ground nearest a target (and the loser having to use their mouth to pull the "pegged" knife out of the earth), but Pop did give me a lesson or two on whittling. My dad's favorite things to whittle were "ball-in-a-cage" and chains. Have you ever seen a chain carved from a block of wood? They are pretty amazing, but with patience and a fair amount of skill they are not particularly challenging to an experienced whittler. The ball-in-a-cage is a little more difficult. If, in your effort to make the ball round, you get it too small, it will fall out of the cage, and you've failed. Unfortunately, getting a lesson and learning to whittle are not strongly correlated in me. I can look at numbers and see patterns, trends, and anomalies, but I can't look at a piece of wood and see the finished product like a whittler.

In the early 70's, the Kenner toy company introduced a sculptor's kit called "Chip Away", promising hours of fun. The premise of the toy was that inside a "block of stone" was a figurine that could be revealed using a toy hammer and chisel. In reality, the "stone" was simply some soft material encapsulating the figurine – no skill required, and no way for you to come up with something different than I.

A lot of people come to God with the notion that they are a "blank slate" and that all they need is to have God add to their life the things they lack, but I tend to think that we are more like a block of stone, and buried deep inside is the masterpiece that the Lord wants us to become. The problem is that a lot of my bad habits, hurts, and hang-ups prevent the God-designed masterpiece inside me from being revealed. Have you ever seen the movie, Shadowlands? It's about a portion of C.S. Lewis' life (portrayed by Anthony Hopkins) when he meets and falls in love with his wife (portrayed by Debra Winger). In that film, he is lecturing a group in London when he says, "We're like blocks of stone, out of which the sculptor carves the forms of men. The blows of his chisel, which hurt us so much, are what make us perfect."

God has already designed us to be the way he wants us to be! We have allowed the things of life to get in the way – attach to us, confuse us, detract us – from being all God wants us to be. And while it's nice to think we can be blank, and God can add to us what he wants, let's realize that what we might need to do is ask God to chisel away those things that hinder us. Not only do I need to think of myself as a sculpture still in need of chisel blows, I also should consider that others around me are in the same position. I don't need to pass judgment on where they need the hammer to fall; I just need to be willing to submit to "The Sculptor." When a lady from our most recent R4G class finished her first non-stop three-mile run, she was so shocked she had completed it. From the beginning, she doubted ever being able to complete the program. My message to her was, "The awesome was already inside you – we just helped it be revealed."

Kent Ogle – *Web City, MO*

James 1:25
But he who looks into the perfect law of liberty and continues in it, and is not a forgetful hearer but a doer of the work, this one will be blessed in what he does.

1 Samuel 16:7
But the Lord said to Samuel, "Do not look at his appearance or at his physical stature, because I have refused him. For the Lord does not see as man sees; for man looks at the outward appearance, but the Lord looks at the heart."

Hebrews 12:11

Now no chastening seems to be joyful for the present, but painful; nevertheless, afterward it yields the peaceable fruit of righteousness to those who have been trained by it.

scripture memorization

Write out the scripture(s) in the space below and recite them ten times.

something to ponder

HOW COULD (OR HAS) THE RUN for God program help(ed) you uncover a strength, ability, or _______ that's been buried deep inside you, just waiting to be revealed?

IS THERE SOMETHING IN YOUR LIFE that "The Sculptor" needs to chip away?

ARE YOU BOLD ENOUGH TO PRAY that you will begin to see people the way God sees them?

HOW DO YOU THINK THAT MIGHT change your perceptions?

running observations by dean

Getting Serious About Recovery

HOW MANY TIMES HAVE WE HEARD some version of the phrase, “It’s not what you say, but what you do, that counts,” or, “Actions speaks louder than words.” We are constantly focused on getting things done to prove our worth and make an impact on the world. There is no question that performance is important, whether considering your job, family responsibilities, or training, but there are times when we get so busy performing tasks that we lose focus on making sure we’re taking the time to prepare to do the right things.

As it relates to running, your body has to have rest in order to continue answering the demands you are putting on it. If you continue to demand more and more every day, eventually your body will rebel and break down physically. The world is full of runners with potential who failed to reach their pinnacle because they did one of two things: 1) They think the phrase “no pain, no gain” is a bunch of hooey and they thought they could get there being comfortable, or 2) They take the phrase “no pain, no gain” literally and think that they should be in pain every day to achieve the highest level of fitness possible. The truth is that the best runners are usually right in the center of these two mindsets. They run hard when it’s time to run hard, and they get plenty of rest in between those hard efforts.

In the long run, hard work pays off, but only if you are smart about the way you apply the effort. When you run, you are creating tiny tears in your muscles. As you rest, your muscles repair themselves to become stronger than they were before the run. If you begin the process of tearing before the repair takes place, it will eventually lead to weakening, and then on to injury. You should always schedule a day off or an easy run the day after a hard effort to allow your muscles time to repair. The older you are, the more time you need to heal. I'm forty-nine and my body needs two days to heal. I have found out the hard way!

What are some things you can do to aid in your recovery? First, stretching after any hard effort will begin the recovery process. When you run, especially when you run hard, your muscles tighten. Taking some time to stretch, post workout, will help to elongate those muscles again. Second, eat something within thirty minutes of working out, but choose what you eat carefully. Eat something low in fat, high in protein and some carbohydrates. Third, make sure you get good sleep and of a duration that is adequate. Everyone's sleep requirements are a little different, so there is no standard, but you know what it takes for you to feel fully rested. Finally, leave time between hard runs. You should not feel sluggish from your last hard effort. For races, a good rule of thumb is to run easy for a number of days equal to the miles in the race. For example, that would be three days for a 5K or two weeks for a half marathon.

In our spiritual life, taking the time to slow down and listen to God is tough. There are so many demands on our time that it can seem overwhelming. Martin Luther once said, "I have so much to do that I shall spend the first three hours in prayer." Like resting from running allows your muscles to rebuild, taking time for God allows your spiritual life to flourish. Without a strong, firm relationship with Jesus, nothing else matters. We have to turn our conventional thought on its head and realize that we can't afford NOT to spend time with Him. Psalm 46:10 says, "Be still, and know that I am God; I will be exalted among the nations, I will be exalted in the earth!" I believe that if we make time to spend with Him, He will provide us with all we need to accomplish all He has for us to do.

- *Your body must rest in order to build the strong muscles, tendons, and ligaments you will need to keep going.*

- *It takes surprisingly few really hard efforts to see improvement in your running. When in doubt, take time to recover instead of hammering your body again.*

- *We have to take time to charge our spiritual batteries. That time includes much more than church one or two days a week. It's all about our relationship with Jesus Christ.*

____

____

____

29
Week

26.2 miles and fixing your eyes on Jesus

I HAVE NEVER REALLY BEEN MUCH of an athlete. I never hit a home run in little league. I never caught a touchdown pass in high school. And yet, here I am in my mid-50s, and by God's grace and strength, I recently ran my second marathon of

26.2 miles.

Running has become my "empty nest" hobby. The Apostle Paul talks a lot about running races in the New Testament. He notes the value of physical training, but he says that spiritual training is more important as it prepares us for the life we live in the full presence of Jesus for all eternity. There are so many different stories to tell and analogies from my experience in running this recent race that parallel life. Two are quick to come to mind. The first is this: Nobody gets up and decides they are going to run a marathon today and does it. It takes time. It takes training. It takes discipline. There were many weeks during the winter when I had to get out there and run 20+ miles on a Saturday morning and this particular winter was not kind to runners, even south Texas runners. Some of those Saturdays were very cold and rainy, but it didn't matter. I ran the distance that my coach told me to run. Sometimes it was really fun! It was delightful, the wind at my back and not a care in the world. Other mornings it was wet, and I bundled up and slogged through the miles. Some days I carried specific and heavy burdens to the Lord in prayer with every mile, but it was all discipline, training, and preparing my body for the grueling task of running for five hours on the first Saturday in April. Because I did three full months of training and stuck to the race day plan, I achieved my goal! I beat the five-hour timer with six minutes to spare!

In life, there are some seasons that may feel like training runs, where it's cold and rainy, difficult or challenging. Finances are a mess. The marriage is rocky. Health is compromised. The job is stressful. Children are childish. In order to succeed, we must keep getting out there, week after week , season after season, and by doing so, our perseverance leads to strength.

Jamilia Williams ran in the 2015 Irving Marathon carrying the American Flag on April 4, 2015. Jamilia Williams is from Las Cruces, New Mexico. She runs for Team Red White and Blue, an organization that honors our military veterans and wounded warriors. During my marathon she carried a four-foot-tall American Flag for the whole 26.2 miles! With the flag high above the runner's heads, I could easily see her for miles and miles from my spot at the back of the pack. In fact, I chased her for 20 miles. When I finally caught up to Jamilia, I thanked her for being an inspiration, without even knowing it. I told her how I kept seeing those Stars and Stripes ahead and how it egged me on to run faster and run harder. She told me she carries the flag for those who are no longer able to do so. I shared with her the verse in the Bible from Hebrews 12, where we are encouraged to "fix our eyes on Jesus." I mentioned how when I fixed my eyes on her flag way out in front of me; I was also calling out to Jesus to give me strength for the next mile. We ran back and forth for about a mile and, since I was following my training plan and drinking lots of water, I had to duck into the port-o-let at Mile 22. When I came out, she was out of reach again. She finished five minutes ahead of me.

The passage from Hebrews 12 reads, "Therefore, since we are surrounded by such a great cloud of witnesses, let us throw off everything that hinders and the sin that so easily entangles. And let us run with perseverance the race marked out for us, fixing our eyes on Jesus, the pioneer and perfecter of faith. For the joy set before him he endured the cross, scorning its shame, and sat down at the right hand of the throne of God. Consider him who endured such opposition from sinners, so that you will not grow weary and lose heart." (Hebrews 12:1-3 NIV)

I'm certain there are many who are just like Jamilia Williams. You lift high the flag of Jesus, and of your churches, and of your schools, neighborhoods and of your families. You are such an inspiration to many and you don't even know it. You serve, you love unconditionally, and you keep doing so every single day, even when it's not easy. Like running a marathon, life is not a flat, open course. You have had to run up some very long hills when you just didn't have the energy to do so. You may have been weary-eyed and physically spent, but because you are keeping your eyes fixed on Jesus, you are making it, and you are inspiring many! I'm here to tell you, when you are going through your rough struggles, make a plan, stick to it, keep trusting

God, and you will make it.

How am I so sure? First of all, because I made it! The marathon I ran had a long, slow, uphill climb around Mile 23, and yes, by that time in the race, my running form did not look much like it did at Mile 3. It was grueling, but once I made it to the crest, those final miles were downhill and rewardingly easy. I had trained well, so I finished well. I eventually sprinted the last 100 yards.

What's another reason we all can run well? The Hebrews 12 text says it is because those who have gone before us are cheering us on. Parents, grandparents, and friends- they have set the example for us. They have encouraged us to always keep the banner of our King Jesus raised high, and by their inspiration and example we can accomplish much. We can steadfastly accomplish the goal and the vision God has set before us. So, my call to you is to keep on running the race. Keep praying. Keep training. Keep listening to what Jesus has to say to you. Keep His vision set before you, and as He leads, be courageous and follow. Be obedient. I believe the best part of this race is ahead of us. I also believe when you train, stick to the plan, and keep your eyes on Jesus, you will finish the race as I finished my last marathon - with great strength, a fist pump or two, maybe even with tears running down your cheeks and with great joy!

Rich Ronald – *San Antonio, TX*

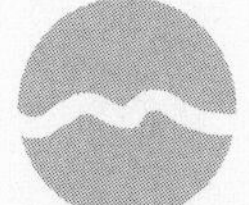

get in the word

Hebrews 12:1-3

Therefore we also, since we are surrounded by so great a cloud of witnesses, let us lay aside every weight, and the sin which so easily ensnares us, and let us run with endurance the race that is set before us, looking unto Jesus, the author and finisher of our faith, who for the joy that was set before Him endured the cross, despising the shame, and has sat down at the right hand of the throne of God. For consider Him who endured such hostility from sinners against Himself, lest you become weary and discouraged in your souls.

1 Timothy 4:7-8

But reject profane and old wives' fables, and exercise yourself toward godliness. For bodily exercise profits a little, but godliness is profitable for all things, having promise of the life that now is and of that, which is to come.

2 Timothy 1:7

For God has not given us a spirit of fear, but of power and of love and of a sound mind.

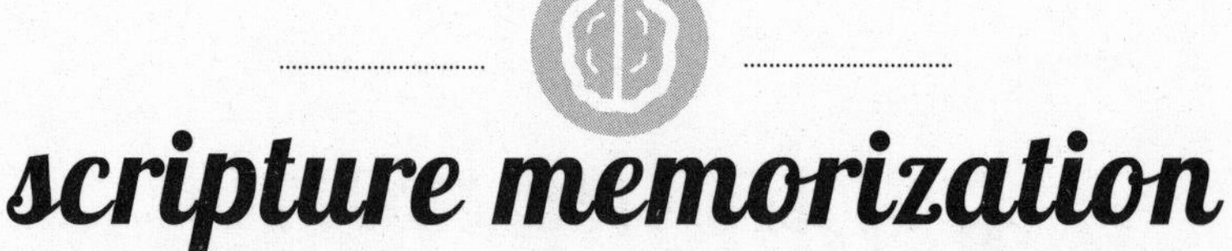

Write out the scripture(s) in the space below and recite them ten times.

___

___

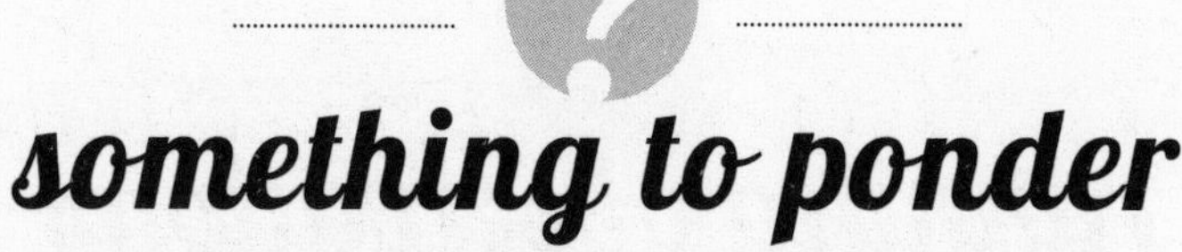

WHEN HAVE YOU SEEN THE BENEFIT of discipline?

HAVE YOU EVER SET A BIG goal and then achieved it? Was there someone who helped you? How did they help?

DESCRIBE A TIME WHEN YOU FACED an incredible challenge and you overcame by the power of discipline, training, making a plan and keeping your eyes fixed on Jesus?

running observations by dean

Metamorphosis

METAMORPHOSIS IS DEFINED AS: A MARKED change in appearance, character, condition, or function. Isn't that what we're looking for? Running does all of those things! If you're a new runner, maybe you are really focused on appearance, trying to lose weight, to become healthier. Or, maybe you have been running for a while and have noticed that the more you run, the better your character becomes. You tend to be more relaxed and more confident. And we're all trying to get to a better condition, whether you're a newbie or a seasoned runner, we're all trying to get lighter, slimmer, or faster. Being a runner means functioning better in every aspect of your life. More than just running better, being more alert and alive in everyday life is a huge benefit of running.

As runners, we're like Monarch butterflies, either working toward a complete transformation or working hard to keep moving forward, making progress. Monarchs begin as plain, not so attractive creatures, that crawl around on their bellies. They work through stages to eventually become beautiful creatures that soar with ease. When we are new to running, or coming back to running after a long absence, that transformation is what we are searching for. However, unlike the butterfly who transforms by being still, we change by being active. We are constantly bombarded with advertisements for things that will make us fitter or healthier by being minimally active. Take this pill, try that new apparatus that only takes ten minutes a day, or try the magic diet that will have you shedding pounds faster than a wrestler trying to make weight. But, the truth is, there are no healthy shortcuts. That's why we're runners.

It doesn't stop there for Monarch butterflies. Each winter they migrate thousands of miles from the northern United States and southern Canada southward to Florida and Mexico. But they have been transformed into bodies that are fit for the journey! Once you have run long enough, and chosen to eat better, your body is fit for even greater things. After your journey changes from crawling on your belly to soaring thousands of miles, it makes all that work worth it!

One other thing that Monarchs teach us is self-preservation. Did you know that they taste horrible? They taste bad so that predators will leave them alone. Isn't it amazing how God created them? Don't forget that you have to take precautions to avoid going back to the larval state. Regular cross training, stretching, and proper diet will help you remain a butterfly. Don't forget to continue to do those things that keep you where you want to be.

God wants us to be transformed. 2 Corinthians 5:17 says, "Therefore if any man be in Christ, he is a new creature: old things are passed away; behold, all things are become new." That sounds like the definition for metamorphosis to me! But, the journey doesn't stop there. If we have truly been transformed, we will want to do all we can for the cause of Christ. 1 John 3:9 says, "Whoever has been born of God does not sin, for His seed remains in him; and he cannot sin, because he has been born of God." If you haven't chosen to go through that transformation, what are you waiting for? If you have, find strength in 1 John 3:9.

- *Metamorphosis is defined as: A marked change in appearance, character, condition, or function. It is what all budding runners strive to achieve.*

- *Like the Monarch butterfly, transforming our bodies through the benefits of running will allow us to soar to places we have never seen.*

- *God wants us to be transformed through Jesus so that we can reap all the benefits of being part of His kingdom.*

sticky notes

broken into pieces

IN MARCH 2005, AT THE AGE of 33, I was in an accident that turned my life upside down. I took a horrible fall. To some, that should have been no big deal, but I had a birth defect that I was not aware of. I started going to a chiropractor who was pulling my leg down, trying to get my hip to stay in place, but instead, my hip was crumbling into pieces. As my hip crumbled, nerves were pinched; I was in pain and suffered from depression. The pain had gotten so bad that I was not able to bend over to tie my shoes, or dress myself and the swelling became a big problem with my health.

My husband could not deal with the issues that came from the accident and walked away. I went to several doctors who offered no hope. One suggested I sit in a wheelchair for the rest of my life which was not an option for me. I prayed and I prayed.

In the summer of 2006, someone suggested an orthopedic doctor who did a great job with my total hip replacement surgery. After weeks of physical therapy and an amazing church family to support me, God healed me. He picked me up when I felt the road ahead was dark and lonely. I am now walking because God answered my prayers.

I have completed six 5ks and one 5 mile race last summer. I have completed four 5ks this year with a goal to accomplish more. I try to do as many races as possible, because I know it was only by the grace of God that I am able to get up and walk, each and every day. I want to share with everyone that my God is amazing..

Sometimes we need to be knocked down to be able to look up and talk to God. Through this journey, He taught me patience. Everything happens in God's time, not ours. I am very thankful God was listening and picked me up, put me back on my feet and gave me the ability to share His grace and healing with others.

Kathy Lawrence – *Morgantown, KY*

get in the word

1 Thessalonians 5:17
Pray without ceasing.

Matthew 19:26
But Jesus looked at them and said, "With men it is impossible, but not with God; for with God all things are possible."

Hebrews 12:1b
And let us run with endurance the race that is set before us.

scripture memorization

Write out the scripture(s) in the space below and recite them ten times.

____

____

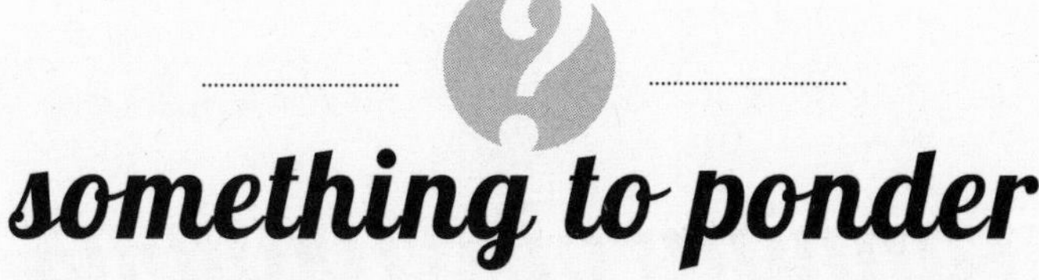

something to ponder

WHEN LIFE is filled with trials, it's easy to ask "WHY ME?" The harder question is "WHY NOT ME?"

WHY DO you think God allows trials to happen to us?

WHY IS it important to learn that God's timing is perfect and ours is flawed?

running observations by dean

He Knows My Name!

MY WIFE, DEBBIE, AND I JUST returned home from a great experience in central Ohio. We filled three eventful days in Columbus at the Capital City Half-Marathon and Expo meeting new friends and listening to some great stories. On race morning we were sure to be near the starting line so we could cheer for over fifty Run for God participants. We positioned ourselves about three hundred meters down the road from the starting line and looked for the Run for God logo as the runners filed by in large groups that were released every couple of minutes. We shouted support for all we could pick out of the crowd.

Once all the waves had been released, we walked a few blocks away to a point where we could see all the runners passing by again. We positioned ourselves at a point where the half marathoners were close to nine miles into their journey, while the quarter marathoners were at five miles and the 5K runners were at two miles. Again, we were looking specifically for Run for God logos, but we were cheering for all who came by us whether they were running or walking. We began to let everyone know just how awesome they were for getting out of bed, toeing the line, and having the determination to reach the finish line, some running as fast as they could and others attempting to cover a distance they had never covered before. Their goal was to cross the finish line.

It was fun to be an encouragement to those who passed by. I would shout, "You look great, keep going!" I would see smiles on many faces as they heard my words, which only encouraged me to be louder for the runners behind them! I would hold my hand out and get some high fives as they passed by. I would comment on their shirt or costume as they came by, which broadened the smile a little more.

But the widest smiles were reserved for those who heard their name. The race organizers had seen to it that everyone's name was printed on their bibs. For those I could read as they raced past, I would call out a name and many of them would look at me with an expression of, "He knows my name!" Of course, I wasn't quick enough, nor can I see well enough, to call out all the names as they came by. I remember one lady holding her bib at an angle to get me to call out her name, but I had already focused on the one beside her, and it was too late by the time I had realized it. I missed her, but fortunately, Debbie, who was thirty meters up the road, recognized what had happened and called her name out as she passed by her. People love hearing their names called out!

And then there were the people towards the back of the pack who were struggling to get through. You could look at the faces and tell which ones were full of doubt. I reached out, grabbed theirs hands as they passed by, put my other arm around them as I moved with them and told them at close quarters that they were going to finish what they started and that God would help them to the finish line. One lady stopped to give me a great big sweaty hug on her journey. It was awesome!

Whether you are walking with Christ or not, He is calling your name. He is there to give you a hug and doesn't care how sweaty or how much doubt, pain or grief you carry with you. He is along every part of the course we have chosen to run and is willing to pick us up and carry us all of the time. One of my favorite verses of scripture is Joshua 1:9: "Have I not commanded you? Be strong and of good courage; do not be afraid, nor be dismayed, for the Lord your God is with you wherever you go." It doesn't matter what course you are on, or where you are on your journey towards the finish line, Jesus is wherever we look for Him, even in the darkest corners. He's calling out your name just waiting for you to acknowledge Him so that He can embrace you and be with you on your life expedition!

- *He knows your name!*

- *Take some time to be an encourager at a local race. The runners really appreciate the support.*

- *Don't be afraid to be loud and a little crazy when supporting runners. Personal recognition means the most.*

- *Look for Jesus on your journey. He is constantly there and eternally willing to encourage us along the way.*

sticky notes

running to God in the

darkest moment of my life

ALMOST THREE AND A HALF YEARS ago, my life was turned upside down. I got a phone call that I wish for no one to ever have to receive. My father called to tell me that my twin brother had passed away. He had a seizure that took his life. I remember feeling completely hopeless, scared, and empty. I felt so many horrible feelings, but in the midst of it all, I remember having a wonderful comfort in knowing that Alex was right where he should be.

He was where we all strive to be at the end of our lives. Alex lived a very full life in only 25 years (2 weeks shy of our 26th birthday). He was an amazing man of God. He recently had taken on running as one of his many activities. He had participated in sprint triathlons, and was in the best shape of his life. As a way to keep his memory alive, my family decided to organize an annual memorial 5k. We have raised money for a scholarship to be given in his name at the college he attended. We had great success in our first two years. However, I stood at the finish line, very overweight, clicking the button as I watched the runners come in. After our last race, the very next day, I decided things were going to change. It was time to make Alex proud, and take care of the body that God has given me.

I started walking and counting calories, and then we started Run for God at my church. I'm a long way from my goal, but I am running. I will run **I'mx's Memorial Race** in April 2015. I have been amazed at the amount of scripture that references our spiritual walk as a race. I hope my story can inspire someone to get out there and get moving. Remember that God wants us to enjoy this life, and being healthy is so much more enjoyable.

Abby Vaughab – *Davisville, WV*

2 Timothy 4:7

I have fought the good fight, I have finished the race, I have kept the faith.

Acts 20:24

But none of these things move me; nor do I count my life dear to myself, so that I may finish my race with joy, and the ministry, which I received from the Lord Jesus, to testify to the gospel of the grace of God.

Jeremiah 29:11

For I know the thoughts that I think toward you, says the Lord, thoughts of peace and not of evil, to give you a future and a hope.

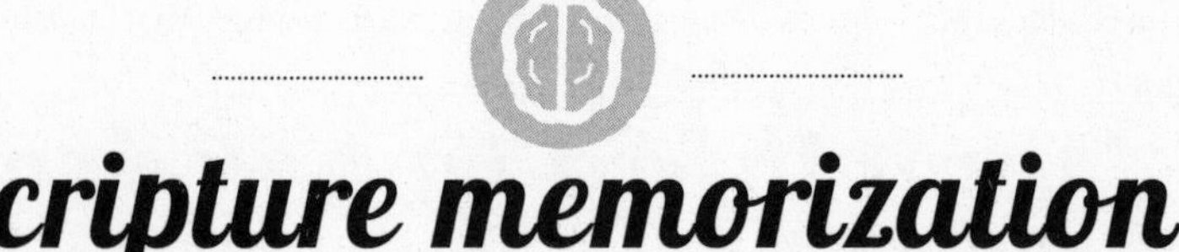

Write out the scripture(s) in the space below and recite them ten times.

something to ponder

WHERE WOULD you be if you surrendered to God a year ago?

CAN YOU really get out of this mess on your own?

running observations by dean

Leaving the Sedentary Lifestyle

FINAL DECREE OF CHANGE

This cause is heard on this day, January 1, 2016 in support of the person we will call Runner. Also appearing before the court is the defendant, Inactivity. Runner has waived her right to an attorney and pleads her case for divorce from Inactivity.

THE COURT FINDS THAT:

That the pleadings of Petitioner are in due form and contain all the allegations, information, and prerequisites required. The Court, after receiving evidence, finds that it has jurisdiction of this case and the parties and at least ten years have elapsed since the date the suit should have been filed. The court finds that the Petitioner and the Defendant, Runner and Inactivity, have been domiciled together for a period of time to be considered fundamentally united. All persons, including friends and family of the Petitioner, having any interest whatsoever in this case have been notified.

FINDINGS OF FACT AND CONCLUSIONS OF LAW

1 COMPETENCY: The Petitioner is competent to plead her case and is of sound mind (finally).

2 ABUSE: The Petitioner has been abused by the Defendant and forced to comply with stringent demands of indolence. The result of these demands is excessive weight, poor health and lowered self-esteem.

3 Mental anguish: The Defendant has mentally manipulated the Petitioner and has influenced her children, Motivation and Determination, to have nothing to do with her. Being the rightful parent of her children, she should have unfettered access to them.

4 – Influence of Friends and Family: The Defendant has controlled the perception of Friends and Family to believe that Inactivity is all the Petitioner needs to subsist, accepting the sedentary lifestyle as a normal part of the Petitioner's life. It is clear to the court that this lifestyle has led to the aforementioned Abuse.

IT IS ORDERED AND DECREED THAT:
Runner, the Petitioner, and Inactivity, the Defendant, are no longer associates and that the association between them is dissolved on the ground of an unhealthy relationship.

IT IS ORDERED AND DECREED that, Runner is granted sole and exclusive custody of Motivation and Determination. Inactivity has no interest or rights to them heretofore.

IT IS ORDERED AND DECREED that Runner retains possession of Positive Thinking, Self-Esteem, Happiness, Courage, Dignity, Inspiration, Joy and Positive Energy.

IT IS ORDERED AND DECREED that Inactivity retains possession of Doubt, Self-Pity, Cowardice, Laziness, Depression, Insecurity, Discouragement, Hopelessness, Pessimistic, and Negative Energy.

IT IS ORDERED AND DECREED that this is a final judgment, for which there is no return and no obligation to the former lifestyle. This judgment finally disposes of all claims of both parties. This judgment is, however, appealable.

Wouldn't it be great if it were that easy? Although it may not be that easy, it is that simple. You can make up your mind at any time to change the direction of your life. The difficulty lies in the day to day decisions to keep that promise. If you struggle with finding motivation to keep running, think of it as a contract between you and your new lifestyle. You don't want to let your children, Motivation and

Determination down, do you?

2 Corinthians 5:17 reads, "Therefore if anyone is in Christ, he is a new creature; the old things passed away; behold, new things have come." When we become His, we put away the old self and focus on the new person Paul speaks about. However, the Bible also tells us that there will be obstacles to overcome. When you make a decision to change your life, there is excitement in that decision, but soon, doubt creeps in because there is difficulty in staying on the path. When we are saved by His blood, we don't become perfect, and we don't give up every time we reveal our imperfections. So, why would we give up on running, cycling, swimming, weight lifting, Zumba class, or any other form of exercise just because we fail once or twice? It is a constant struggle to keep the words of our decree of divorce from an unhealthy lifestyle. But we know, with Christ, all things are possible!

- *Deciding to change your lifestyle is the easy part. The difficulty comes in the day to day battles fought to stay on the right track.*

- *Although it is not easy to say focused on good health with all the temptation and distractions, it is a simple concept, like a contract.*

- *When we become Christians, we become new and our old lifestyle passes away. But we will always have to battle our imperfect selves to be what God wants us to be.*

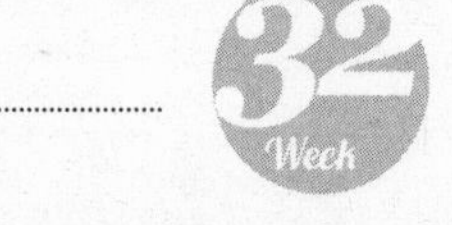

a reason to run

I HAVE BEEN GOING TO CHURCH my whole life, and I always thought that as long as I was good and believed in God that I would go to heaven. I believe in God, but I wasn't that interested in going to church. I was born on January 16, 1985, in Kansas City, Missouri, and suffered from Fetal Alcohol Syndrome. By the grace of God, I was adopted by two loving people and became the youngest member of the family. In 1991, I was diagnosed with ADHD and my parents enrolled me in an elementary school specialized for kids with learning disabilities. As I got older, I started learning about God and that He sent His Son Jesus to die on the cross for all our sins, including mine. When I became a teenager, I started to fellowship with other Christians and realized how important it is to surround myself with people who love the Lord. I gave my heart to Jesus when I was thirteen.

In the spring of 2003, I suffered a stroke, due to a hole in my heart, which required surgery to fix. My whole left side was paralyzed, and I lost most of my peripheral vision. After a couple of hours, the stroke resolved on its own without rehabilitation; however, my peripheral vision never came back, which led to much depression and anger. My mom and I talked about it, and she reminded me that there are a lot of people in situations that are far worse than mine. After some time, I started to come around and God gave me the strength to get through it. Later that year, I experienced pain, stiffness, and flare-ups throughout my body. One morning I had a flare up in my back and was admitted to the hospital and was diagnosed with Rheumatoid Arthritis. I was worried that this disease would cripple me for life, but my arthritis doctor placed me on medication and said that the prognosis is excellent.

When I was a kid, I would often watch infomercials about kids living in poverty and wanted to do something to help. So I decided to become a child sponsor through World Vision. Over the years, I've developed a passion for running and decided to use my passion to glorify Christ by raising for Team World Vision through the marathons that I run. So far, I've run six marathons and participated in other races, as well. Running for Team World has been one of the things that I'm most proud of in my life. I have three athletic goals that I want to accomplish. I want to run The Boston Marathon, The TCS New York City Marathon, and eventually complete an IRONMAN Triathlon. I don't know how people get through tough times without turning to Jesus? What I do know is that Jesus will get you through the worst times in your life.

Lori Ramsey – *House Springs, MO*

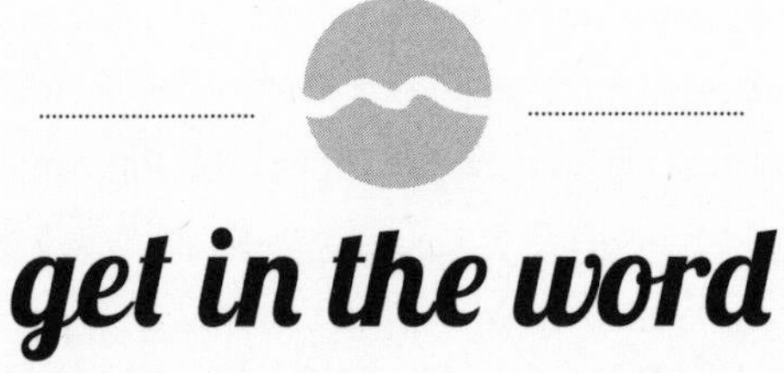

get in the word

2 Peter 1:3
As His Divine power has given to us all things that pertain to life and godliness, through the knowledge of Him who called us by glory and virtue.

Philippians 4:13
I can do all things through Christ who strengthens me.

1 Corinthians 9:27
But I discipline my body and bring it into subjection, lest, when I have preached to others, I myself should become disqualified.

scripture memorization

Write out the scripture(s) in the space below and recite them ten times.

something to ponder

WHY DON'T people turn to Jesus in their time of desperate need?

___

___

___

___

WHY DON'T people want to know about Jesus?

___

___

___

___

WHY DO people blame Jesus for their problems?

___

___

___

___

running observations

by dean

It's All Connected

APPARENTLY, I'M INSANE. I BASE THAT on the fact that I keep doing the same thing over and over and expect different results. We all know we have to do something different when an injury occurs, but runners are a hard-headed bunch. You don't believe me? Ask any orthopedist and he will tell you that talking to a runner about taking time off is like talking to a wall. I'm sure I'm not talking about you. Let's say I'm referring to "other" runners. As it turns out, I happen to be one of those other runners. Oh, I have changed plenty over the years and have mellowed, even become much smarter about my training, but I still have a way to go. I have recently fallen off the wagon.

I am sitting right now with ice on my heel because I have had plantar fasciitis for a couple of months. It would have been healed by now if I had taken it more seriously when it first cropped up, but I didn't, despite the fact I have been through it before. How did I contract this dreaded malady? It showed up because I had a tight hamstring that forced me to change my stride. So where did the tight hamstring come from? That began as a pain in my hip that caused me to favor one side as I ran. So the pain the hip just showed up one day, right? No, it began with a tight IT band. Should I go on or have I made my point?

When we don't care for a pain related to our running, it will either get worse, or it will show itself somewhere else. All of our muscles, tendons, ligaments and bones work together as we run and there is little margin for error in your stride. If one problem crops up and you alter your stride, chances are that another pain will show up because everything is connected. The old song we used to sing, "The hip bone connected to the leg bone, the leg bone connected to the knee bone, etc." makes a lot of sense now. I always say, "Soreness is okay, pain is not." I just don't listen to myself very well.

And here's the worst part; just because you have pain doesn't necessarily mean you have to stop running altogether. I have found over the last week that my pain is subsiding by just cutting back the mileage and running easy. It was that simple the whole time! Did I mention that we runners are a stubborn bunch? I share this to say, "Don't be like Dean. Be smarter!" When you have pain, do something about it. That may mean something as simple as applying ice after every run, or it may mean taking time off from running, but take action. In my case, I have felt like I'm a little behind in training for an upcoming triathlon, so I didn't want to back off. Now I will start that race with the fear that my foot will cause me problems on the run. My fault, I know better.

As a Christian, I know all that matters is my relationship with Jesus. I tend to make living life more complicated than that, as many of us do. We often seem to think that we have to follow a bunch of rules to be good Christians, but Jesus boiled it all down to this in Matthew 22:37-39: "Jesus said to him, 'You shall love the Lord your God with all your heart, with all your soul, and with all your mind.' This is the first and great commandment. And the second is like it: 'You shall love your neighbor as yourself.'" Love is the answer. Jesus is telling us that, if we love God and everyone around us and show them our love, everything else will fall into place. So why do we make it so complicated by arguing about the minutia of our faith?

- *All of our muscles, tendons, ligaments and bones are linked together. When something goes wrong in one area, it is bound to affect others.*

- *If we react to pain at the first sign, we can avoid some long layoffs.*

- *It's simple: Love is the answer.*

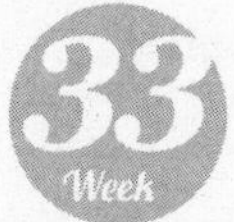

running God's race

"RUNNING GOD'S RACE" AS A RUNNER and Christian school teacher, I thought I knew what it meant to "run God's race." This teacher had a lot to learn.

This year's 2014 C.I.M. (California International Marathon) will mark my 25th marathon. Somewhere between this race and my first marathon in 2009 on the streets of San Francisco and Golden Gate Bridge, a transformation occurred. I went from being a middle-aged teacher, mom, and wife just wanting to say she finished a marathon, to a child of God just wanting to hear her Father say, "A race well run!" However, the journey to this mindset has been challenging and not a flat course.

After a few PRs, I allowed myself to think that maybe, just maybe, I could qualify for Boston. Boston? I didn't even know what the Boston Marathon was six years ago. It might as well have been the Olympics. The problem with setting a goal as high as Boston is that anything short of it soon becomes failure. Whether you're eighteen minutes away (as I currently am) or eighteen seconds away, it's still failure, or so I thought.

I had two key epiphanies this year. The first one came during a 19-mile training run. The TobyMac song "Eye On It" came up on my iPod Shuffle around mile 16. This was one of my third grade class' favorite songs as we often talked and prayed about keeping our eyes focused on the true prize of running toward God's calling in our lives. Philippians 3:14 even became a class cheer as we reminded each other to "Press on" and keep our eyes on the prize.

On any given run, whether it's training or racing, many prayers emerge. On this particular day, I made the leap from praying to RUNNING WITH GOD. Imagine running with your best friend - you would just talk about what was going on in your life, the highs and the lows, and you would encourage each other when you were tired and ready to call it quits. You would keep running together, and you would just be grateful for the company. Something happened in my spirit that day as I realized I didn't need to keep asking – and sometimes begging – God to help me finish a run. It wasn't that I had lost sight of what this "prize" was in Philippians 3; God showed me that I was trying to get that prize in the wrong way – my way. As I finished this run, chatting it up with my Coach, I felt an overwhelming peace that honestly felt better than any PR I had attained. I could 100% honestly say that "the prize" was spending time with Jesus Himself, not a new personal record or any medal (and I do love cute medals).

The second epiphany came during the Oakland Marathon. I had the privilege of meeting my running hero, Olympic marathoner, and brother-in-Christ, Ryan Hall, at the L.A. Marathon Expo two weeks earlier. I had read his book several times called Running with Joy. Ryan signed my running shirt with the scripture John 10:10 "I have come that they may have life, and have it to the full." This verse was a game changer for me, and God illustrated it right before my eyes beginning at the Oakland Marathon starting corral. This was the first time I had seen mini-bibs on runners with the word "FULL." They were pinned on runners' backs (in addition to the standard size race number on the front) indicating full marathon vs. relay. I had a "FULL" bib pinned on my back as well but thought nothing of it at first. It wasn't until I got in the starting corral that I saw a sea of the word "FULL" before me. Why is this significant? After reading Ryan's book, I had asked God to help me run with the kind of full joy described in his book. I also prayed to experience this "life to the full" in all areas of my life. I realized right before the starting gun went off that I would be staring at the word "FULL" for the entire marathon.

God knows me so well. He knows I need these not-so-subtle reminders to depend on Him and His Word to fuel me from start to finish. This was not an easy marathon, but it was certainly one of the most enjoyable. Driving home from Oakland that day, I realized that marathons are not an end in itself but one leg of an incredible journey. After years of reading, praying, analyzing, and espousing Hebrews 12:1, this marathon was finally my connection: running the race God has marked out for me takes place on a life-long course. I will easily become discouraged or go off-course if I am only focusing on my own short-term plans and goals. Don't get me wrong; there is nothing wrong with short and long term planning. In fact, it is wise and prudent. But I realized somewhere between marathon one and marathon twenty that I had made personal records the end all and reason for my joy.

Irene Tang – *San Ramon, CA*

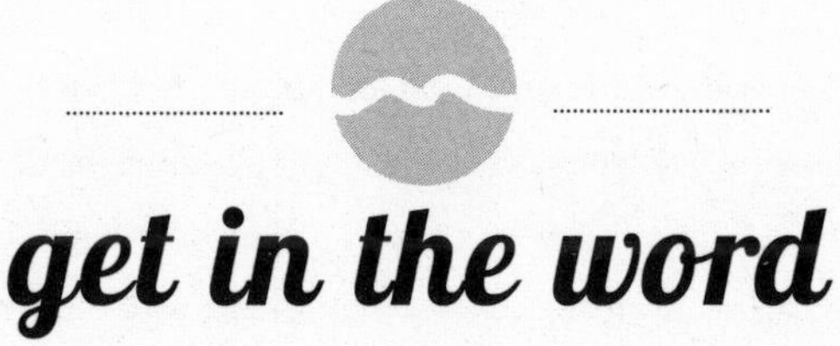

Philippians 4:13
I can do all things through Christ who strengthens me.

John 10:10
The thief does not come except to steal, and to kill, and to destroy. I have come that they may have life, and that they may have it more abundantly.

Hebrews 12:1
Therefore we also, since we are surrounded by so great a cloud of witnesses, let us lay aside every weight, and the sin which so easily ensnares us, and let us run with endurance the race that is set before us.

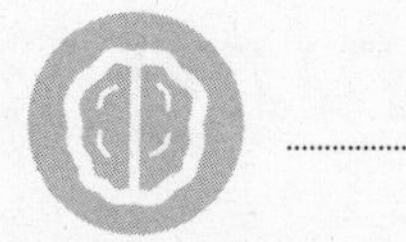

scripture memorization

Write out the scripture(s) in the space below and recite them ten times.

something to ponder

HOW DOES God direct the way we set running goals?

____

____

____

____

WHY DID God use running to connect with Christian living?

____

____

____

____

HOW DO I really know if I am running for God or for myself?

____

____

____

____

running observations by dean

Running and Humor

RUNNING AND HUMOR GO TOGETHER. THERE are a number of funny sayings that are associated with the running community: "Run like you stole something." "Run like someone just called you a jogger." "Worst Parade ever." "Even Chuck Norris never ran a marathon." "In our minds, you're all Kenyans." "May the course be with you." They're funny! Another way to think about it is this: What is a runner's favorite compliment? Answer - "You're crazy!" It's true, isn't it? Running has funny words like "fartlek" and "bonk." And if you're whining a little too much, you just need to "suck it up buttercup" as a good friend of mine would say. When running a race, there is this saying; "My first thought when I start a race: Why am I doing this? My first thought after a race: When can I do it again?" As runners, we have complicated relationships with things like the treadmill. We love it when the weather is bad, but we hate it at the same time! Maybe the fact that we're a little confused adds to the humor!

How many times have you heard the phrase "laughter is the best medicine?" It is a phrase that goes back many, many years and it is as true today as it was many years ago. Laughter produces endorphins which make you feel better, so scientifically, the phrase is correct. Many studies have been done to show that the physical act of laughter will trigger an increase in endorphins, the brain chemicals known for their feel-good effect. Not only do the endorphins make us feel better, but they give a general sense of well-being that has the effect of making us more tolerant of pain, which comes in handy when we run!

Another phrase that is regularly uttered around the running community is "runner's high." So, what is runner's high? Similar to laughter, the body releases endorphins during endurance events. It results in a euphoria that we refer to as "runner's high." For many years, it was thought that these endorphins were part of the body's response to stress; therefore, they would not be found in the brain, but in the bloodstream. The debate went on for thirty years over whether or not there was a "real" runner's high with endorphins being released into the brain. More recently, research has caught up, and now there is proof that running in endurance events does cause the release of endorphins into the brain resulting in a runner's high. The running community knew it long ago, but science just caught up. Interestingly, the studies also confirmed the same thing that laughter showed: The release of these endorphins increased pain tolerance, which explains ultra-marathoners.

Anything that you get excited about has the potential to release endorphins in your brain and make you feel good. Getting excited about the one and only true God can have a very positive effect on your mood. We often look for things to "pick us up" when we are feeling down. Sometimes, all it takes is a little Bible study and prayer time. If you do that, and then go out for a run, and see something funny on the side of the road, you may become overwhelmed by the joy of it all!

- *Laughter produces endorphins that make you feel good.*
- *Running, or any endurance event, can also release these endorphins, which explains the term "runner's high."*
- *Getting excited about the God of the universe is enough to make anyone giddy with excitement!*

sticky notes

running for the prize

JULY 26, 2013, MY 42ND BIRTHDAY, was a day that changed the trajectory of my life. This date marks the day that I signed up for my first 5K. I was scared because I have never done anything like this before. I watch The Biggest Loser every season and admire the contestants running and having fun doing it. My brother-in-law is a runner and has many medals from his races. I always thought to myself that I could do that and could have a display of medals in my house.

Many voices in my head kept telling me that I was too old, too fat, and too out of shape, but the Lord kept reminding me that I was "fearfully and wonderfully made (Psalm 139:14)." God made me for a purpose and that purpose was to run for Him. He gave me a desire to run and get healthy for many reasons. First, running provides me with a chance to spend more time with my Heavenly Father. I talk with Him and He talks to me. Next, running keeps me healthy for my family. My father has diabetes and is not doing well. My mother is his caregiver. I do not want my wife to have to take care of me if I get this illness. I love my wife so much that I don't want to burden her with this.

Now, back to training for my first 5k. I am not going to say it was easy. Some days, I didn't feel like running, but God gave me the strength to keep on keeping on. I got a wonderful app for my phone which helped me train from the couch to a 5k. I trained for three months and was ready for my first 5k.

I was nervous that morning and woke up before my family to pray that God would give me the strength to run the race before me. As the starting gun sounded, I ran my heart out. I ran the course and kept praying that God would be with me. I saw the finish line, and my emotions came over me. I started crying to God that I have done something beyond my own strength. I ran it in 41 minutes, which to me was a good springboard for future goals. After that 5k, I accomplished four more. I trained hard with God's strength. I pushed myself to run a mile without stopping. I did it without any trouble with God's strength. I pushed myself to run two miles without stopping, and I did it again with God's strength. Then I pushed myself to a new level. I challenged myself to run a 5k without stopping like I had done in my most recent 5K. When I was scared that I could not complete this goal, a verse that I wrote on my feet Philippians 4:13, reminded me that I could: "I can do all this through him who gives me strength."

I started the race at a great pace. I kept running the race as God kept talking to me to run for the prize of the finish line. The finish line came into my sight, and I was still running. I completed the 5k in 35 minutes. I praised God that He was there and thanked Him that He will continue to be there as I run the race on Earth. My next challenge God has put on my heart is to run a 3-race challenge (5K, 10K, and half marathon).

Running and training for a race has similarities to running and training for the race on Earth for God. Just as God pushed me to run farther each time, God wants us to push ourselves and step out of our comfort zone in order to grow in our relationship with Him. A race on Earth gives us a medal but God gives us treasures to store in heaven. Paul raced the best race in the Bible, and a verse that God has placed on my heart lately is 2 Timothy 4:7 "I have fought the good fight, I have finished the race, and I have kept the faith." I want to finish the race and get the prize of eternal life with my Heavenly Father.

Brian Tooley – *Hemet, CA*

get in the word

Psalm 139:14

I will praise You, for I am fearfully and wonderfully made Marvelous are Your works, and that my soul knows very well.

Philippians 4:13

I can do all things through Christ who strengthens me.

2 Timothy 4:7

I have fought the good fight, I have finished the race, I have kept the faith.

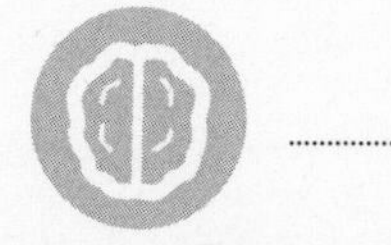

scripture memorization

Write out the scripture(s) in the space below and recite them ten times.

something to ponder

WHY IS God using me?

____

____

____

____

HOW CAN I decipher God's voice in the middle of training?

____

____

____

____

WHAT ARE the similarities of running the race on Earth and for God?

____

____

____

____

running observations by dean

I Used To...

ONE DAY, I WAS BRUSHING MY teeth, and I dropped my toothbrush. I made the comment to my wife, Debbie, "I used to never drop things." I used to be so coordinated. Her response was sympathetic, as it always is, although I deserved different because that was probably the 100th time she had heard that line come from my mouth. I used to be able to do a lot of things I can't do anymore.

I used to run much faster than I do now. Age has slowed me down, and I don't much care for it. I used to be able to get into shape after coming back from an injury in six weeks. Now, it takes six much more painful months. I used to be able to run hard every other day. Now, if I get in two hard runs in a week, I need a full week of recovery. In addition, my body continues to change, and I have to constantly adjust my training to avoid injury. If it sounds like I'm whining a bit, I guess I am.

Alfred Lord Tennyson wrote in his poem In Memoriam, A.H.H., section 27, "'Tis better to have loved and lost than never to have loved at all." The sentiment rings true for me as I think about what I was once able to do, but can no longer achieve. When I look back, I realize that I was fortunate to accomplish what I did. Dwelling on the past can be good or bad, though. I know people who either quit running because of the frustration of slowing down, or cannot let go of the past, always talking about what was rather than what can be. Reminiscing is okay, even fun, as long as we're not obsessive about it.

I have come to realize that looking forward is preferable to looking back. I find that when I look forward, I change my focus to something more in line with reality. I love to get together with old running buddies and talk about what once was, but it's more like looking at photos in an album than trying to relive the past. Today, I think about things I never thought about in the past. I love to cheer for the mid-packers and back-of-the-packers like never before. I have cultivated a deep respect for those who spend more time out on the course than I do. And don't get me started on watching someone finish her first 5K after struggling with the training that leads to the triumphant day. There's nothing better.

Jesus said in Luke 9:62, "No one, having put his hand to the plow, and looking back, is fit for the kingdom of God." Jesus was telling us that once He changes us, we should be focused on spiritual development, never going back to the person we were before. We learned some good lessons in the past, but we should only lean on those lessons inasmuch as they help us to live a God-centered life. The closer I get to Him, the more I realize I'm better than I was but not as good as I'm going to be. I may be slower and weaker physically, but I'll take the spiritual strength of the Lord any day. He is far stronger than I ever was!

- *If you're an aging runner, you were probably faster at one time, and it can be frustrating. If you're not an aging runner, just wait....*

- *Reminiscing can be great as long as we're not obsessive about it.*

- *vWhen we accept Jesus as Lord and Savior, we only look back at the lessons that are valuable to our walk with Christ. We now live in His strength.*

sticky notes

running to win

MY HEART LEAPT WITH JOY AS I read Isaiah 43:18-19 which says to forget everything in my past. Of course, I should forget about past errors and mistakes and press on to run toward what is ahead of me on my narrow way. Yet, I believe these verses also command me to forget even my mountain-peak experiences with God because they are nothing compared to what He is planning to do with my present and my future. The word says He is going to do something new in me, and He has already started. How exhilarating it is to know He truly does have plans to prosper me, to give me a hope and a future. Because of the goodness of God, I want to live my life to glorify the Lord. I want to eat right and exercise, so I can be fit to serve Him the rest of my life. I want to run toward all the plans He has for my future. I want to become all He wants me to be. I want to run in such a way that I might WIN. I want to WIN in my daily walk with the Lord, overcoming all my shortcomings. I want to WIN other people to the Lord by sharing the story of how He transformed me from the inside out. I want to win my eternal salvation, hearing the words from my Jesus "Well done my good and faithful servant."

Xxxxx Xxxxx-*xxxxxxx, xxxxxx*

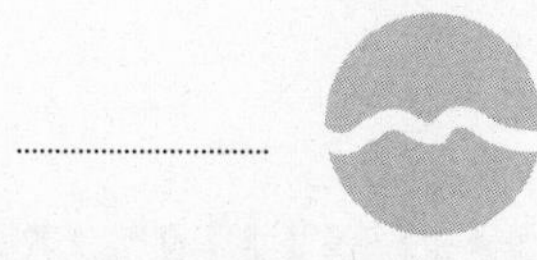

get in the word

Isaiah 43:18-19

"Do not remember the former things, nor consider the things of old. Behold, I will do a new thing, now it shall spring forth; shall you not know it? I will even make a road in the wilderness and rivers in the desert.

Jeremiah 29:11

For I know the thoughts that I think toward you, says the Lord, thoughts of peace and not of evil, to give you a future and a hope.

Philippians 3:13

Brethren, I do not count myself to have apprehended; but one thing I do, forgetting those things, which are behind, and reaching forward to those things which are ahead.

scripture memorization

Write out the scripture(s) in the space below and recite them ten times.

something to ponder

WHAT PAST FAILURES AND MISTAKES DO you need to forget to move toward the Lord's future plans?

WHAT MOUNTAINTOP EXPERIENCES DO YOU NEED to forget to embrace the new work God has started in you?

WHAT DO YOU NEED TO CHANGE to WIN in your daily walk?

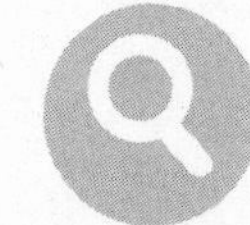

running observations by dean

You Can Restore an Old Car...

THERE'S A SAYING AMONG THE CAR community that goes like this: "You can restore an old car, but it's still an old car." It means that, no matter what you do to something older, you will still have the problems associated with the fact that it has lived past its normal, most useful, life.

When you restore an old car, it can be made to look like new. You can replace all the wearable parts, rebuild the engine, re-upholster the seats, and give it new paint on the exterior. Essentially, the car is new in the same way that a house feels new when you restore it. But what happens with an old car or an old house after the restoration? Things go wrong that wouldn't go wrong with a new car or a new house. They don't have all the gadgets and fancy features of the new model. They're not as comfortable as the new ones, are they?

On the other hand, a classic car is fun to drive. The beautiful lines of the body stir our souls. These cars became classics for a reason! The high ceilings and intricate woodwork of an old house reminds us of the love and artistry that went into them when they were built. In both cases, they remain useful. The classic car gets us from one point to another just like a new car, and when you drive it, heads turn to catch a glimpse. It's not something people see every day, so they're intrigued to see a piece of history traveling down the road.

The most important part of the car is the engine. As long as it will get you from one place to another, everything else is just superficial. Of course, all the other parts are needed to make the vehicle useful, but as long as the engine is sound, the condition of everything else is not critical. The engine may have more weight to carry, and it may not handle as well as a new one, but the engine can overcome those factors.

As we age, we become classics! Sure, we are going to have more problems than younger runners. Yes, we have to spend more time in "maintenance" than our junior counterparts. We may not have fancy gadgets like super-fast sprinting speed, but we still have a working engine! And, although we may have to use that engine to overcome poorer handling and a few extra pounds, we can overpower any negative that age throws our way. We can be unencumbered by the need to compete with the "newer models" because we have already had our time, but when we run down the road, through the trail, or around the track, heads are turning. They're turning in admiration to see the "classic." We're not in the junk yard or parked in the garage to go to waste. If you don't use an old car, rust and rot take it over. We have realized that keeping our bodies moving is the best hedge against old age!

The Bible is as relevant today as it ever has been. Someone once said, "It is more up to date than tomorrow's newspaper." The Bible has been around a long time, but it never gets old. There's no need to restore anything! Isaiah 40:8 says, "The grass withers, the flower fades, But the word of our God stands forever." We're going to get older and our bodies less compliant. We're going to have to work hard to keep it moving, but one day we are going to have a new body and the aches and pains of this world will pass away. The Bible says so, and it stands forever.

- *You can restore an old car, but it's still an old car. You can train an old body, but it's still an old body.*
- *As we age, we become classics. We might have to work harder to keep fit, but it's even more impressive than a young person being fit.*
- *God's word endures forever.*

running for a change

MY NAME IS DANIEL KIEWEL, BUT to most people who know me, I'm D.J. (or when I am in trouble, it is Daniel James). I grew up in Aurora, Colorado, and have a Bachelor's Degree in Technical Journalism from Colorado State University in Fort Collins. The first 22 years of my life in Colorado shaped who I am and my values as a Christian, but if you're looking for the man the Lord has made me into, the first twenty two years becomes the prologue, if you will, to the story - at least when it comes to faith, and to running.

In January 2003, I moved to the region I've called home for the past ten years now, rural west central Kansas (at least, rural by the definition of someone who grew up in Denver). Every step of the way was what the country music group Rascall Flatts calls a "broken road" that led me to where the Lord has brought me now, and while the Lord has used the pain of the first few years in Kansas to shape me, the entire premise of this story is to "press forward", in racing, in faith, and in life, and not to dwell on the past, but keep your eyes focused on the prize that is ahead. This is where we get to the three events that have most impacted and defined who I have become.

In February 2008, I met a wonderful woman, Staci Swartz, who became my wife in July of 2009. She has been one of God's greatest gifts and blessings in my life. In July of 2008, I had a chance to meet Mark Williams, founder of a men's homeless ministry, Prodigal Ministries, through whom I got involved with a group of intrepid souls like myself at Extreme Hope Christian Fellowship (now CrossPoint - Great Bend), where I am still heavily involved today. My running story begins in early 2010 while at a church youth function in Great Bend. Up to this point, you must understand, I despised distance running. My twin sister, Diana, had done it for all four years in high school, competing on our school cross-country team. I just thought they were all insane, but it all changed with an anger-filled, five-sixths of a mile lap around Veteran's Lake in Great Bend, Kansas. This is when the Lord lit the fire within me. I realized how good a run was for relieving stress, and how healthy that could make me if I did it consistently. It would not be until later, though, that I would realize just how profoundly it would impact me, and those around me, spiritually. That is the most important reason for my running, and one huge reason I continue to do it. It has changed my outlook on faith and life entirely.

My first competitive run was in a 6.2-mile (10 kilometer) run in Great Bend, Kansas, my current hometown, the MDA Run, on June 17, 2010. I finished in just over 56 minutes, walking part of the way, but realized then, how much I loved the atmosphere of race day. So, since then, I have competed in numerous 5-k (3.1-mile) and 10k (6.2-mile) races, a 15k (9.3-mile), four half marathons (13.1 miles). Because family is such an important part of this to me, I have been blessed to run with them in many of these races. My wife, Staci, has participated in three of these nine races, and has been one of my strongest supporters in the endeavor. My twin sister, Diana, who I used to think was insane, has been a part of four of them. My father, Jim Kiewel, who has had so much to do with the man that I have become, and the man I most admire and am influenced by on this earth, has participated with us in two of those races. If there is anyone who embodies what it means to overcome great difficulties in life, it is he. I am so blessed to still have him and my mother, Karin, who has been by his side for the last 39 years, both still as a large part of my life. My mom, who has battled rheumatoid arthritis, also competed with us in a race, as well, the first of several "Family Affair" Eisenhower Marathon in Abilene, KS April 2012. All this is only the beginning - now I look to the present and focus on the goals the Lord has placed in my heart for my life.

April 2014 marked a monumental occasion in my life. I was able to accomplish the monumental goal of finishing my first full 26.2-mile marathon. As of this writing, in November 2014, I am planning to run a second in Oklahoma City in April 2015. More importantly, though, I have been blessed to connect with several friends who share the same passions for running, and for pursuit of a relationship and service of the Lord, Jesus Christ. As I grow, I am also increasingly seeing opportunities to use this gift and passion the Lord has given to impact the world around me, and am seeing just how much this gift is able to do just that. I have had opportunities to become an active part of our community-running group, as well as part of the fundraising group, CareRunners, to be able to run for local charities. The older I get, and the more I run, the more I learn that running, and life, is an ever-changing process of learning and growth. There are always goals to reach, hurdles to overcome, and finish lines to cross. The only true destination for it all is Heaven, and an eternity with Jesus Christ. Writing and distance running are just two tools He has given me to reach that destination, and to help others reach it, as well. Until we reach it, the journey is never truly complete.

After all of this, I have become a firm believer that nothing is impossible through the strength of our Lord and Savior, Jesus Christ, if you have the strength, and determination to pursue what He has called you to do. I am also living proof that no one is beyond hope of transformation because of the love of Christ, regardless of one's past mistakes. You are not defined by your past, but by the hope of Jesus Christ you have inside you. This is me, and I am glad you have decided to join me on this journey of running, and more of faith and perseverance. I hope you will stick with me, and that it might inspire you to pursue the "out-of-reach" dreams of your own! May the Lord bless and keep you, and in Jesus may you find the "hope and future" for this life and beyond!

Daniel Kiewel – *Great Bend, KS*

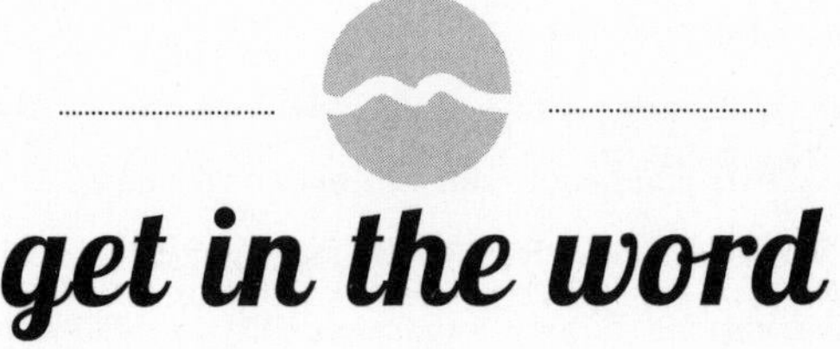

get in the word

Philippians 3:12

Not that I have already attained, or am already perfected; but I press on, that I may lay hold of that for which Christ Jesus has also laid hold of me.

Jeremiah 29:11

For I know the thoughts that I think toward you, says the Lord, thoughts of peace and not of evil, to give you a future and a hope.

Psalm 62

Truly my soul silently waits for God;
From Him comes my salvation.

He only is my rock and my salvation;
He is my defense;
I shall not be greatly moved.
How long will you attack a man?
You shall be slain, all of you,
Like a leaning wall and a tottering fence.
They only consult to cast him down from his high position;
They delight in lies;
They bless with their mouth,
But they curse inwardly. Selah
My soul, wait silently for God alone,
For my expectation is from Him.
He only is my rock and my salvation;
He is my defense;
I shall not be moved.
In God is my salvation and my glory;
The rock of my strength,
And my refuge, is in God.
Trust in Him at all times, you people;
Pour out your heart before Him;
God is a refuge for us. Selah
Surely men of low degree are a vapor,
Men of high degree are a lie;
If they are weighed on the scales,
They are altogether lighter than vapor.
Do not trust in oppression,
Nor vainly hope in robbery;
If riches increase,
Do not set your heart on them.
God has spoken once,
Twice I have heard this:

That power belongs to God.
Also to You, O Lord, belongs mercy;
For You render to each one according to his work.

scripture memorization

Write out the scripture(s) in the space below and recite them ten times.

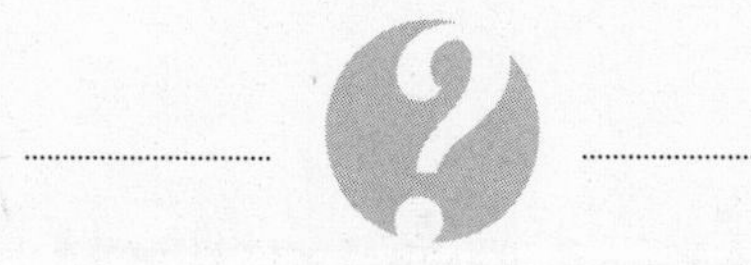

something to ponder

HOW ARE you using your gift of running to build up lives in the community around you?

HOW HAS running deepened your understanding of your relationship with Jesus Christ?

____

____

____

____

HOW HAS running brought you closer to family and friends?

____

____

____

running observations by dean

Running Surfaces

IS RUNNING BORING? I HAVE HAD many conversations with non-runners who believe the monotony of running is too much to bear. However there are a number of things that enable us to make it more exciting. I'd like to focus on one of those things; the type of surfaces we use in our training.

It has been my experience that most runners have a preference of one surface over others. My favorite surface is the road. I like the smoothness of the road that enables me to focus on thoughts about things other than running. The sure footing of the road imparts more speed to my runs which always makes me feel better about my fitness level. In addition, the constantly changing scenery is something that makes the road more interesting than some other options. It helps me keep some focus on being connected to the neighborhood, giving me opportunities to get to know neighbors I may not have met otherwise. Running on the road is probably the most used surface by veteran runners, but not so much by those who are newer to the running community. If you are a little skittish about getting out on the roads, it doesn't take long to get more comfortable. Perhaps the greatest benefit of the road is that it begins at the end of the driveway, making it easily accessible.

I know many runners who prefer the trails. Being out in nature is always rewarding. The peace, quiet and solitude it offers are irresistible. Sometimes there is interaction with wildlife. Although most of that interaction is interesting and positive, like seeing deer scamper through the woods, squirrels running up trees, or rabbits running across the trail, there are other, less positive wildlife sightings, like animals without shoulders; snakes! Of course, some people love snakes and look forward to those sightings. Running the trails also requires more concentration than other surfaces because of the unsure footing. You have to constantly look out for rocks, roots or other impediments to your stride. Trails tend to be hillier and slower than other surfaces. For many runners, that is the draw. They like the challenge it imposes on the body and they enjoy it more as the difficulty level increases.

Many beginning runners start their newfound exercise on the track. The track offers the easiest running and the least distractions of any running surface. There are no hills, no rocks, you won't get lost, and you're always close to the start, which can be good or bad. If you have difficulties with your run, it is much easier to stop. If you have an injury or a thunderstorm blows in, you are close to the car and a much safer environment. Of course, it also makes it easier to stop because it gets hard, which is not always good. For some, the temptation is too great! Of course, the track is a great place for speed workouts and many veteran runners find themselves at the track often to hone their fitness and speed.

The treadmill represents the final major running surface. It provides variety in that you can vary speeds and incline, but the scenery never changes. Many people will catch up on the news or other television programs while running on the treadmill, providing an opportunity to kill two birds with one stone. In addition, the treadmill is great for bad weather days. Conditions are always consistent. The treadmill is also a good tool for harder workouts. Running interval sessions on treadmills is a little different from running hard on the track, but can provide the same benefits.

There are other running surfaces, like the beach, for instance, that make it fun to be a runner. You just have to be careful. I remember thinking it would be cool to run barefoot on the beach once. And, that's how many times I have done it, once! I didn't stop to think that the effect of running barefoot on sand would be similar to running on sandpaper. It made the next day's run a little tough on my tender feet!

Just as there are many different surfaces on which to run, there are many ways to serve the Lord. We all have spiritual gifts, those things we prefer to do and areas where we excel, but there are many ways to please the God of the universe. I believe having a consistent ministry focus is important, but I also think it is a good idea to venture out of our comfort zone a little and into areas that help us to grow. Do you know what your spiritual gifts are? Do you use them regularly? What can you do to venture out and grow in your ministry?

- *One of the beautiful things about running is the variety that it provides in running surfaces and scenery. Don't be afraid to venture out onto all of them to find your favorite!*

- *Be careful when trying a new running surface. They all have a different effect on your body. Proceed cautiously.*

- *Take time to understand what your spiritual gifts are so that you can be most effective in your worship and can have the most positive impact on those around you.*

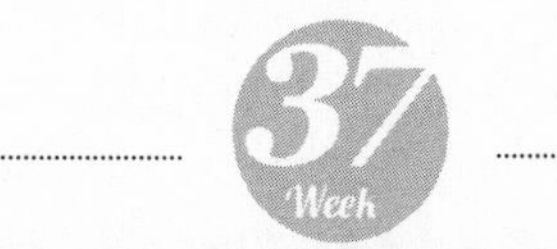

run with God

I MUST ADMIT THAT, ALTHOUGH MY faith is a big part of my life, I don't usually express it within the running community. When I was asked to teach a lesson for our Wednesday night adult Bible study, choosing any topic that related to faith and Christianity, the topic of living a healthy lifestyle immediately came to mind. I thought it only natural that I write a perspective on this topic and share it with you, my running friends, as well as my friends from my Wednesday evening Bible study.

Throughout my years of running, I have come to realize that running has played a part in making my faith stronger. It seems only natural that this might happen for runners or any other active individual. Some situations in running create a more natural tie to spirituality than others.

For me to remain excited about running over the years, I have had to mix up my workouts a little. Speed work, recovery runs, tempo runs, hill training, track work, running on city roads, running on rural roads and trail running are just a few of the ways I maintain variety in my running. All variations of running help me to see God in my life, especially those that allow me to take in the natural beauty of our earth. I am not here to say that every run that I have completed over the last decade has intensified my spirituality, but I can't help but feel that pushing my body to its limits, feeling the rhythm of my heartbeat and working up a sweat helps me feel a sense of accomplishment that might bring me closer to and appreciate my maker. Certainly, not just the workout itself, but also the reflection during and after each workout has always been something that has allowed me to appreciate a higher being.

Many individuals who are not active, might think it too daunting of a task to improve their health and fitness, but for those of you who can remember your fitness level for your first run and your fitness level now, there is no doubt that it is never too late to improve your own health and fitness. It doesn't matter how old or young you are, you can always find a way to improve your fitness level whether it be with brisk walking, cross-country skiing, biking, swimming, running or whatever aerobic activity you choose. The key is to start slow and increase your effort as time pushes on. In my experience, I have come to realize that the human body is like a rubber band. You can't necessarily put limitations on what your body can do, but if you start out slow and keep working, you can stretch your body's physical abilities, beyond those imaginary lines you thought that you could never cross. Patience and perseverance are crucial for this to happen. Nothing happens overnight. Not only will becoming more active and deliberate in your dietary intake improve your physical well being, but it will also boost your mental and emotional resolve.

There are many studies that show a link between physical activity and mental and emotional health. Physical activity will not only improve your physical fitness, but also has the potential to strengthen your mental function, boost your self-esteem and enhance your spiritual well being. So where then does a spiritual being begin this journey into making his or her temple more fit? Pick an activity that you might enjoy. You might enjoy doing this activity alone or you might find it easier to share it with a friend. Start out slow and make it part of your routine. You should try to be aerobic at least three times a week to maximize your potential. If you are able to build it into your routine of at least thirty minutes three times a week, you will find that it will be more of a natural part of your life and not such a chore. You may also find it helpful to keep a log of your exercise. It might be a source of motivation for you to see where you started and how far you have come.

It's important to remember that exercise is just part of the equation. You must be wise about your diet. Eat sensibly and in moderation. Also allow yourself ample rest and recovery time. With a health and fitness routine in place, chances are you will not only extend your life, but also improve the quality of it, as well. The emphasis for this particular article has been to take care of your body for God, but don't ever forget that you are also doing this for yourself as well as your friends and family. If you can find it in you to stay healthy and active, you might provide the motivation for someone else to do the same. This is especially important for our future generations. With childhood obesity running rampant in our country, modeling how to lead a healthy lifestyle can establish important habits for our children. If you are a parent or a grandparent, your daily healthy routines have more of a positive influence on your children or grandchildren than what you realize. What better way to be a role model than through living a healthy, active lifestyle? Not only will running be positive for you and your relationships with friends and family, but it will also allow you to strengthen your bond with God. KEEP RUNNING!! Until next time, this has been just another runner's perspective.

Gale Fischer – *Battlecreek, MI*

get in the word

1 Corinthians 6:19-20

Or do you not know that your body is the temple of the Holy Spirit who is in you, whom you have from God, and you are not your own? For you were bought at a price; therefore glorify God in your body and in your spirit, which are God's.

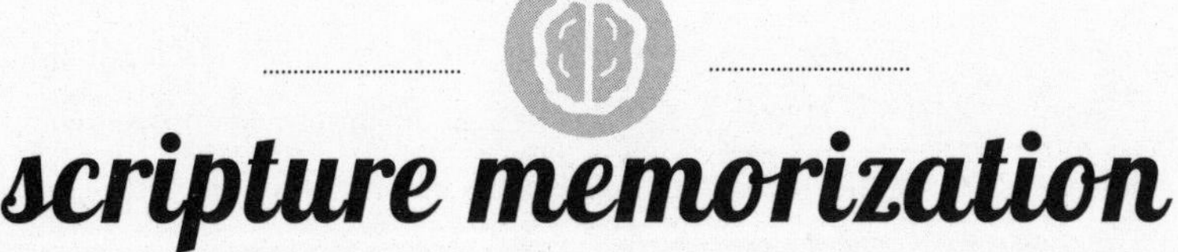

scripture memorization

Write out the scripture(s) in the space below and recite them ten times.

something to ponder

HOW DO your physical, mental and emotional experiences work together to boost your spiritual well being?

____

HOW CAN your running bring others to know God?

WHAT WILL strengthen your relationship with God more, running alone, running with others or will both work equally?

running observations by dean

Train Up Children in the Way They Should Go

THERE ARE SO MANY MORE OPTIONS available to kids these days than when most of us were growing up. I remember making up a game I could play by myself where I would toss rocks in the air and hit them across a pond with a stick. That kind of activity may exist today, but I would think it is few and far between. I found running because it was one of the dozen or so options available to me when I was young. Video games were played in game rooms and weren't anything like what is out there today, and sports like Archery, among others, weren't anywhere close to the radar. There were some bad things to get involved in, but fortunately, I found positive things to occupy my time, for the most part. There are still bad things out there today, so it is important that we focus children on positive activities. With the choices today, it should not be a problem to keep kids busy in those events.

Running is an excellent activity for children for many reasons. To begin with, teaching them to run enables you to share the positive physical benefits of exercise with them. Building good, healthy habits at an early age will only increase the chances of living a lifetime of good health. In addition, we also know that there are great mental benefits to running in the form of confidence and better self-awareness. When kids are runners, they tend to hang out with other kids who are participating in the same great activity. I don't know if there is a study somewhere that bears this out, but in my experience, runners are usually better students than other athletes or average students. Hanging out with smart kids can only benefit our children.

Running is something a child can continue to do for an entire lifetime. Football players don't have that opportunity. Also, almost anyone can run track and cross country in school. In most schools, there are no tryouts and cuts. If a student wants to run, she can participate. There are few opportunities in sports where those at the lower end of the talent spectrum can participate with the highly talented. All inclusive sports, like cross country, are great activities to keep kids away from all the distractions and negative things in which they could be immersed. There is a lot to be said for keeping kids busy!

Last, but just as important, the running community outside of school sports is very supportive of everyone who wishes to participate. Being around fun, healthy, positive and encouraging people is a goal that all caring parents want their children pursuing. What other sports can be enjoyed together across all ages as well as running? And, think about the positive feelings they will have when they finish the local 5K and look back at all the adults finishing behind them.

We are all familiar with Proverbs 22:6: "Train up a child in the way he should go; even when he is old he will not depart from it." Getting them on a good foundation by encouraging them to participate in a lifetime activity, like running, will yield positive attributes. Just don't forget that the passage in Proverbs is also referring to spiritual guidance. Children are our responsibility. Even if you don't have children, you can be a positive influence through your support and encouragement. Psalm 127:3 says, "Behold, children are a heritage from the Lord, the fruit of the womb is a reward." Let us all nurture and encourage them!

- *Running is a great activity for children because it surrounds them in a positive culture.*

- *Running is a lifetime activity to be enjoyed and shared across generations.*

- *Children are blessings from God. Ensuring that they develop positive habits is Biblical.*

sticky notes

38
Week

passing it on

I WAS ONCE UNINTERESTED IN RUNNING. I didn't believe in God. I was broken hearted. God restored and saved me over the years. I began to quit some bad habits and began to want to change. A fitness instructor believed in me. She pushed me harder and farther than I ever thought I could go! Now, with two sprint triathlons and many 5ks under my belt, my desire is to glorify God and worship Him with my life. One of the ways that I do that is by encouraging and believing in others that have never run a 5k. With the Run for God program as a key to success, I believe with God, all things are possible. There may be some hills in life and hills on the road. The hills are hard. The trials of this life are hard, but there in the hills, God helps us and we push on strong for him. We come out on the other side giving him fame. We are victorious through Jesus!

Amy Levins – *Sutton, MA*

get in the word

Proverbs 3:5-6

Trust in the Lord with all your heart, and lean not on your own understanding; in all your ways acknowledge Him, and He shall direct your paths.

Psalm 147:3

He heals the brokenhearted and binds up their wounds.

Matthew 28:20

Teaching them to observe all things that I have commanded you; and lo, I am with you always, even to the end of the age." Amen.

scripture memorization

Write out the scripture(s) in the space below and recite them ten times.

something to ponder

HOW HAS God pushed you through to reach victory?

HOW CAN you help someone else believe it is possible for him or her to overcome obstacles?

HOW DOES God want to use you to help someone come to Him?

running observations by dean

Running Efficiency

EVERYTHING IN LIFE BECOMES MORE EFFICIENT with time. If you are old enough to remember vinyl albums, you recall that there was enough room on each side of an album for four or five songs. It meant that you would get a maximum of about ten songs on one album. And think about the space the album occupied! When compact discs came along, they were smaller and held more songs. Today, I can hold an MP3 player in my hand that contains a pick-up load of vinyl albums! Not only that, if I want the latest Jeremy Camp album, I can purchase and download it in seconds from my couch. It sure beats getting in the car to go to the record store! How efficient the music industry has become.

If you have ever watched world class runners on television, the first thing you notice is that they don't look like you and I when they run. Why? For the most part, they have worked all of the inefficiency out of their running form. You may not be able to run like them, or even look like them when you run, but you can become a more efficient runner, too.

First, stride length is important. If your foot strikes the ground too far out in front of you, it's like putting on the brakes with every stride. You won't feel yourself slowing down with each stride, but if your foot lands too far in front of your center of gravity, it is happening. If you can see your toes way out in front of you each stride, you may want to try focusing on keeping your feet under your hips a little bit more.

Your cadence is the number of times your feet strike the ground expressed in time, usually per minute. Your run cadence may change based on the speed you are running, but not nearly as much as you would think. Famous coach, Jack Daniels, studied Olympic athletes running middle and long distances and found that nearly every one of them had a cadence of right at 180 strides per minute. When you are racing, this is probably a good target. If your cadence is less, you may be over-striding. When you're out for a normal training run, you may find that your cadence is lower, but it should still be above 160, or 80 per leg. Of course, there are adjustments for height, but again, not as much as you would think. If your stride is different from these suggested cadences, it's okay, but by measuring your cadence, you can learn and experiment with what works best for you.

Improving the position of your body is another way to increase efficiency. When you run, make yourself tall and don't slouch your shoulders, but keep your shoulders relaxed. Your hips should be slightly forward so that you are bending forward from your ankles. It is important to understand that the angle is not from your waist. Leaning forward by bending at the waist puts extra stress on your legs and back. Also, as you are running tall, be sure you are not bouncing. Again, it is extra energy, wasted.

Your arms should provide stability while your body rotates, but that rotation should be minimal. Keep your elbows bent at 90 degrees, and don't let them cross your center line. Arms are used more when sprinting and running uphill because they help provide lift. Don't forget to take advantage of that lift when running uphill.

Your legs should finish the push and then follow through to the next step fluidly. The leg pulls through more easily when the knee is bent. If you keep your leg too straight, you are using more energy than you need.

Over 2,000 years ago, there was a system of sacrifices, rules and ordinances to follow, and a priest to intercede between you and God. It was a difficult process to follow, but it was the only way to show God your willingness to be His child. When Jesus went to the cross, it all changed. There is no more need for animal sacrifices, tedious rules to follow and a priest to talk to God for you, because Jesus provides all of that for us. Romans 5:8 says, "But God demonstrates His own love toward us, in that while we were still sinners, Christ died for us." He paid for our sins and is the link between us and God. Our salvation became so much more efficient when Christ died for us!

- *We may not be able to run like the Kenyans, but we can adopt some of their more efficient ways of running.*

- *Working on your stride length, cadence and your body position can help you run faster and prevent injury.*

- *Jesus provided a more efficient way to the Father when he died on the cross for our sins.*

sticky notes

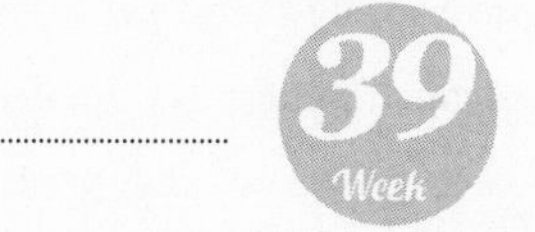

running: a quiet calm

I FEEL A QUIET CALM INSIDE me right now as I reflect on the events of July 2014. If not for love, courage, faith and all of the prayers from our loved ones, I never could have survived the horrifying experience alone. We were NEVER alone.

It was a sunny, hot Monday morning in the Bahamas. The bright sun shining through the windows made me want to jump out of bed and go for a run as I did the day before. God didn't let me run on this day though as my husband calmly told me he needed an ambulance because he thought he was having a heart attack. I ran to the front desk of the condo complex asking for help for my husband and to please call an ambulance. A registered nurse was staying in a condo just a couple of doors down. She gave my husband an aspirin and held his hand while we waited for an ambulance to come.

We barely made it to the hospital. I was standing in the ER, only a few feet away from my husband, when the curtain was drawn as I heard the words "code blue" and "clear". Then I heard it again and again. I thought he was gone; however, it wasn't his time. My husband wanted the doctors to stabilize him and then fly him to Miami to the Cleveland Clinic. The doctors looked at him and told him, "We have 30 to 90 minutes to put a stent in you or you will be dead." My husband then said, "Do what you have to do," and with God's guidance, the doctors worked quickly to put a stent in his heart, as I waited motionless and scared.

Thinking back, I cannot even remember how I started to tell family back in the States. Every time one of our loved ones wanted to give us a hug, a total stranger would approach me and hug me in the waiting room, and pray with me, and I would soon pass that hug to my husband. The next day, I quickly worked to get my daughter and my niece back home, safe and sound. They are two very brave girls. It was a relief when they told me they were home. My husband would not be flying home any time soon unless we were to take an "air ambulance", which is basically an ICU in an airplane. So began my journey to start making arrangements for this to happen.

I would take a cab back-and-forth from the condo to the hospital because they would not let me stay at the hospital. At one point, the doctors told me that he had developed some pneumonia. Now, I really had to get him home in a hurry. I took a cab back to the condo and packed up our suitcases. I had been communicating with an insurance agent about flying my husband home via air ambulance. I went to bed to try to rest.

Around midnight, I received a text saying it could happen the next day. I immediately got back up and made little tags out of paper with our address and taped them to three suitcases. In the morning I had to ship the suitcases home, because I knew there would only be room for a backpack or two on the plane. I left the condo that morning hugging everyone as they prayed for my husband and me to have a safe flight home.

Things did not happen as quickly as I thought they would, and I ended up coming back to the condo to eat one more meal later that night as our plane was scheduled to leave at 2:30 in the morning. I was allowed to stay in the hospital waiting room until the plane would arrive. My husband had been doing well and talking, but was told that intubation would be necessary to fly home. The pressure from the plane ride could possibly cause problems with his breathing, and it would be very hard to intubate in the air, so he agreed.

The plane ride was scary; we had a full medical team of one doctor, one respiratory therapist, and a registered nurse. The oxygen tanks were not working correctly at one point, and they had to use a bag to get my husband his oxygen and because he was not sedated, he was able to cooperate and time it just right. My husband was brave and strong and determined. God had brought us this far and carried us the whole way; I knew in my heart we would make it home.

We landed at approximately 6:45 AM. We were transported to a local hospital of our choice by ambulance. The medical team at the hospital was wonderful and started testing and x-raying him immediately. The x-rays showed no sign of pneumonia. There WERE dark patches and splotches on the x-rays in the Bahamas, and they had told me it was common when you're filled with fluids after surgery for that to happen, but it was all gone now. On the third day, after returning home, I decided I needed to keep training for the half marathon. I knew as, long as my husband was still in the hospital, he was safe. Once he came home, however, I felt very different about going for a run. I was afraid of what might happen if I left him alone for even half of an hour.

Praying about my dilemma helped immensely. I now know that there are certain things we just have to give to the Lord. When worry, stress or a particular problem arises, it's best to say to the Lord, "Please deal with this for me. You can handle it much better than I." A sigh of relief will wash over you if you just give it to the Lord. I found peace in going for my runs while leaving my husband home alone. I knew he was in good hands. I ran my first half marathon, and during my race, I would stop for a beautiful scenic picture, and even post it on a social media site. My friends would comment, "Are you running or taking pictures?"

I thoroughly enjoyed my first half marathon; I did not put an emphasis on time, but on taking in all that God had put in front of me. My husband is a walking miracle. I am very blessed to still have him in my life. The doctors in the Bahamas, told us to come back and WALK through the front door to say hello someday! All Praise to God.

Robin Gilliam – *Strongsville, OH*

get in the word

1 Peter 5:7
Cast all your care upon Him, for He cares for you.

Deuteronomy 31:6
Be strong and of good courage, do not fear nor be afraid of them; for the Lord your God, He is the One who goes with you. He will not leave you nor forsake you."

2 Timothy 4:7
I have fought the good fight, I have finished the race, I have kept the faith.

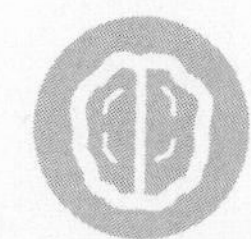

scripture memorization

Write out the scripture(s) in the space below and recite them ten times.

something to ponder

DO WE have any control of our lives?

DOES GOD keep us connected through strangers?

CAN WE give God our burdens and feel relief?

____

____

____

running observations by dean

Running Clothes Don't Make the Runner or Passion Over Fashion

SOME PEOPLE SPEND A LOT OF money on running attire and there's nothing wrong with that. If you are always at the front of the running fashion crowd, you can skip the next four paragraphs if you like. I have something to share with the rest of the pack.

Okay, so here's the deal; you simply do not need fancy clothes to be a runner. While good running shoes are important, all other extravagant running equipment is non-essential, even your clothing. It is one of the beautiful things about our sport. Someone once told me that the reason soccer is so big throughout the world is that it is inexpensive. You need a ball, a few willing participants and a relatively flat area. Dirt is okay! Running is the same way which may explain why it is so big in countries like Kenya and Ethiopia.

For some, there is a worry about what others will think if you don't dress up to their standards. The truth is, for the most part, runners are not very judgmental. Wearing less fancy clothing is kind of like eating a hamburger with ketchup oozing out the side. There may be someone who thinks it's sloppy, but they're probably not going to say anything, and they undoubtedly won't give it a second thought. As long as you're enjoying the burger, running, don't worry about what others are thinking. If you don't have the money, or simply choose not to spend it on running attire you will still gain full acceptance from the running community. If there is someone who views you as less than a "real" runner, you don't really want to hang out with them anyway (but you may want to pray for them!).

Your basic needs are a pair of shorts, a shirt and socks, with appropriate undergarments. The shorts should definitely be made from a synthetic material, like polyester or nylon to keep you as dry as possible and prevent chafing. Most people today prefer the same materials for shirts, although for years it was thought that there was nothing better than a cotton shirt. I just like mine to be comfortable. Some people spend a lot of money on socks. I have found relatively inexpensive running socks to be perfectly adequate for me. It may depend upon the combination of your particular feet, your shoes and your running tendencies as to whether or not you can get by with a less technical sock. If you want to splurge somewhere, I would think socks would be the most advantageous place to do it.

Don't be afraid to try off brands. Ninety five percent of my runs are completed wearing a store brand of shorts for which I pay less than fifteen dollars a pair. I wear t-shirts from races, and I just told you about my socks. There are runners out there with a higher sense of fashion, but there aren't many with a higher sense of passion, and I think it's passion that counts!

When it comes to your clothing, it's really just a shell. It's what people see. The true runner is on the inside, under the clothes. In the same way, we can trick people into believing we are someone we're not by showing them a façade that looks good, while we are much different on the inside. God knows who we are on the inside.

You can wear all the fancy clothing you want, but it won't get you through your next challenging race. You'll be exposed if your training has not been adequate. John 3:19-21 says, "And this is the condemnation, that the light has come into the world, and men loved darkness rather than light, because their deeds were evil. For everyone practicing evil hates the light and does not come to the light, lest his deeds should be exposed. But he who lives by the truth comes to the light, that his deeds may be clearly seen, that they have been done in God." Eventually, we will all be exposed by the light of Christ. It's up to each of us to make sure that we present a pleasing view to Him when the time comes.

- *You don't have to spend a lot of money on clothing to be a runner.*

- *Don't worry about what others think of your clothing. It's the passion inside that will make running most enjoyable for you.*

- *Just like the clothes don't make the runner, our outward appearance doesn't mean anything to a righteous God, unless it is accompanied by a pure heart.*

sticky notes

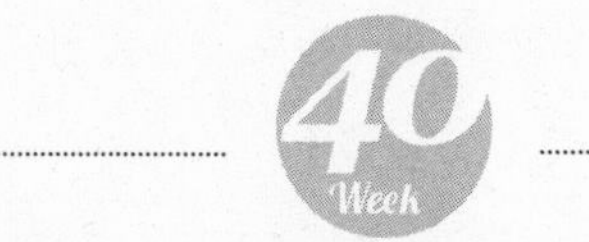

putting faith in action

I HAVE BEEN A CHRISTIAN NOW for a little over five years. I began running last year and immediately loved the sport. We have a group at my church that runs together at many local 5k events. I discovered the Run For God program while searching on the Internet. After thinking and praying about it, I decided to purchase the 5k instructor's edition. Not knowing what was to come, I began studying it myself. I was praying and leaning toward letting our youth pastor at church teach Run For God to us. Well, God's plan was different. After conflicting work schedules and doubts about even doing Run for God, I began running and praying for God to do His will in my life. I became the instructor with a class of 48 for week one.

We are in week eight and have planned our first Run For God 5k at church in October. Trusting God and learning how important faith in myself is through Him taught me everything. Not only is my running stronger, but also everyday struggles tend to work themselves out easier with God. Many of my classmates share the same story. Hebrews 11 provides many examples of faith and actions taken from that faith. Philippians 4:13 reminded me that God is my strength and everything comes from Him. He broadened my understanding of truth through Him. While running, He gave me strength when I felt I couldn't run any more. I have seen God lift others in our class while running, as well. I needed the Run For God 5k program in my life, and His timing of leading me to the course was in His perfect plan.

Craig Walters – *Laurel, MS*

get in the word

Hebrews 11
Now faith is the substance of things hoped for, the evidence of things not seen.
2 For by it the elders obtained a good testimony.
3 By faith we understand that the worlds were framed by the word of God, so that the things which are seen were not made of things which are visible.
4 By faith Abel offered to God a more excellent sacrifice than Cain, through which he obtained witness that he was righteous, God testifying of his gifts; and through it he being dead still speaks.
5 By faith Enoch was taken away so that he did not see death, "and was not found, because God had taken him"; for before he was taken he had this testimony, that he pleased God.
6 But without faith it is impossible to please Him, for he who comes to God must believe that He is, and that He is a rewarder of those who diligently seek Him.
7 By faith Noah, being divinely warned of things not yet seen, moved

*with godly fear, prepared an ark for the saving of his household, by
which he condemned the world and became heir of the righteousness
which is according to faith.
8 By faith Abraham obeyed when he was called to go out to the place
which he would receive as an inheritance. And he went out, not
knowing where he was going.
9 By faith he dwelt in the land of promise as in a foreign country,
dwelling in tents with Isaac and Jacob, the heirs with him of the
same promise; 10 for he waited for the city which has foundations,
whose builder and maker is God.
11 By faith Sarah herself also received strength to conceive seed, and
she bore a child when she was past the age, because she judged Him
faithful who had promised.
12 Therefore from one man, and him as good as dead, were born as
many as the stars of the sky in multitude—innumerable as the sand
which is by the seashore.
13 These all died in faith, not having received the promises, but
having seen them afar off were assured of them, embraced them and
confessed that they were strangers and pilgrims on the earth.
14 For those who say such things declare plainly that they seek a
homeland.
15 And truly if they had called to mind that country from which they
had come out, they would have had opportunity to return.
16 But now they desire a better, that is, a heavenly country.
Therefore God is not ashamed to be called their God, for He has
prepared a city for them.
17 By faith Abraham, when he was tested, offered up Isaac, and he
who had received the promises offered up his only begotten son,
18 of whom it was said, "In Isaac your seed shall be called,"
19 concluding that God was able to raise him up, even from the dead,
from which he also received him in a figurative sense.*

20 By faith Isaac blessed Jacob and Esau concerning things to come.
21 By faith Jacob, when he was dying, blessed each of the sons of Joseph, and worshiped, leaning on the top of his staff.
22 By faith Joseph, when he was dying, made mention of the departure of the children of Israel, and gave instructions concerning his bones.
23 By faith Moses, when he was born, was hidden three months by his parents, because they saw he was a beautiful child; and they were not afraid of the king's command.
24 By faith Moses, when he became of age, refused to be called the son of Pharaoh's daughter,
25 choosing rather to suffer affliction with the people of God than to enjoy the passing pleasures of sin,
26 esteeming the reproach of Christ greater riches than the treasures in Egypt; for he looked to the reward.
27 By faith he forsook Egypt, not fearing the wrath of the king; for he endured as seeing Him who is invisible.
28 By faith he kept the Passover and the sprinkling of blood, lest he who destroyed the firstborn should touch them.
29 By faith they passed through the Red Sea as by dry land, whereas the Egyptians, attempting to do so, were drowned.
30 By faith the walls of Jericho fell down after they were encircled for seven days.
31 By faith the harlot Rahab did not perish with those who did not believe, when she had received the spies with peace.
32 And what more shall I say? For the time would fail me to tell of Gideon and Barak and Samson and Jephthah, also of David and Samuel and the prophets:
33 who through faith subdued kingdoms, worked righteousness, obtained promises, stopped the mouths of lions,
34 quenched the violence of fire, escaped the edge of the sword, out

of weakness were made strong, became valiant in battle, turned to
flight the armies of the aliens.
35 Women received their dead raised to life again. Others were
tortured, not accepting deliverance, that they might obtain a better
resurrection.
36 Still others had trial of mockings and scourgings, yes, and of
chains and imprisonment.
37 They were stoned, they were sawn in two, were tempted, were
slain with the sword. They wandered about in sheepskins and
goatskins, being destitute, afflicted, tormented—
38 of whom the world was not worthy. They wandered in deserts
and mountains, in dens and caves of the earth.
39 And all these, having obtained a good testimony through faith, did
not receive the promise,
40 God having provided something better for us, that they should not
be made perfect apart from us.

Philippians 4:13

I can do all things through Christ who strengthens me.

Psalm 119:32

I will run the course of Your commandments, for You shall enlarge my heart.

scripture memorization

Write out the scripture(s) in the space below and recite them ten times.

something to ponder

WHY IS it so hard to trust in faith?

WHERE DOES our faith come from? Why?

WHAT HINDERS us from obeying the truth?

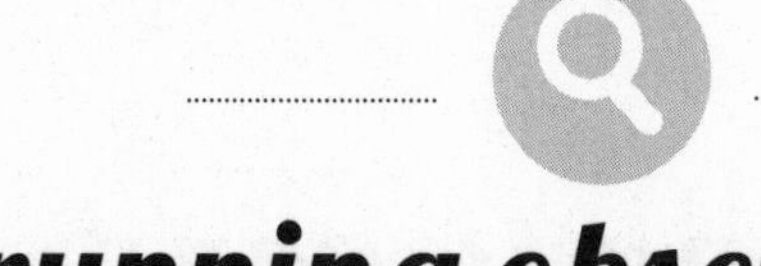

running observations by dean

I Once Was Blind, But Now I See

I REMEMBER THE DAY I LOOKED through my first pair of glasses. I was fifteen years old and had my vision checked because my performance on the baseball field had declined. I was a pretty good hitter when I was fourteen, but the following year I began to strike out a lot. Although I had always had trouble hitting a sharp, breaking curve ball, I never had difficulty with a fast ball, until then. I couldn't understand why I wasn't hitting the ball because I knew I was swinging in the right place. But, I wasn't, obviously! The doctor told me that my vision was poor, and I ordered my new glasses. The next week, before I put them on, the optometrist asked me to look out the front window of the store and across the street at some signs. I could make out the outline of the signs but could not read any of them. I placed the glasses over my eyes, and it was like I was introduced to a whole new world! I could read the signs! I had no idea that my vision was so poor.

There are many people, who would love running, but have never tried, or if they have, they didn't go about it the right way. The cliché, "If you ever see me running it's because something is chasing me," is one we have all heard many times. We grew up with PE teachers and coaches using running as a punishment for doing something wrong. We have been led to believe that running is unpleasant and is to be endured rather than enjoyed. When I tell people I enjoy running, many think I'm crazy, and a few want to book me for treatment immediately.

Most people look at running as something physically difficult. While it is hard to begin running, and there are days when it is all we can do to keep going, there are many days when it feels great. Of course, the problem with that assertion is that you have to do a lot of running to arrive at a point when it is easy. The overwhelming feeling of beginning makes it difficult to see the rewarding days over the horizon. Think back to when you started running, or you were coming back from an injury. It was difficult, wasn't it? The difference is that we know what the end result of the hard work looks and feels like, so it is much easier for us.

The problem is that non-runners simply do not know what they are missing. They have never felt the benefits of better sleep. They've never known the effortless glide of an easy run on a day when everything is just right. They've never experienced the feeling of going to the doctor for a check-up knowing that your blood pressure, cholesterol and weight are going to register on the positive end of the scale. They've never crossed a finish line after months of muscle firming, weight-shedding work with arms raised in conquering victory!

So, when our non-running friends say, "I don't even drive that far" after we tell them about our long run over the weekend, just smile and tell them your car's not that reliable anyway. We have to understand that they have no appreciation for what we do, because they can't see the whole picture. They recognize the hard parts but fail to grasp the rewarding consequences of what we do. Point them to a Run for God 5K Challenge class and, if they are ready, the can catch a glimpse of what you have! The only way they'll understand is to live the experience.

In the same way, our friends who have never experienced a life changing relationship with Jesus Christ do not understand how rewarding our lives become once we begin our walk with Him. They recognize the part where we give up things they believe are fun, or stimulating. They fail to comprehend the meaning of Philippians 4:6-7, "Be anxious for nothing, but in everything by prayer and supplication, with thanksgiving, let your requests be made known to God; and the peace of God, which surpasses all understanding, will guard your hearts and minds through Christ Jesus." They cannot appreciate the security of knowing that God will direct our paths when we rely on Him in all we do. The Great Commission compels us to share those feelings with them. The Holy Spirit will take it from there!

- *Our non-running friends cannot understand the positive effects of running.*

- *We can sympathize with non-running friends if we think back to when we first began running.*

- *We are all sinners. It should be easy for us to understand why our lost friends have difficulty comprehending the awesomeness of God, because we were once there ourselves. We can only help them understand by allowing the Holy Spirit to change their lives, just as He has ours.*

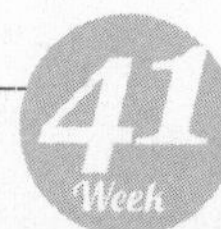

leave earthly judgments at the side of the road

I AM THE ULTIMATE JUDGE AND you are well loved by Me. The world may judge your body; I do not. Your body is a gift, your feet a moving force. Run for Me and I will lead you to a place of great light.

Oftentimes, the world urges you to look a certain way. Society's signals, signs and messages insinuate that your body is not acceptable, as it has been created, as I designed you to be. If the world judges you, then it also judges Me. Allay your anxieties and rest in the knowledge that I have sculpted you with great Love. I am the Potter, you are the clay. My Hands have molded you with exact precision. Your beauty and your worth do not come from this world; they were given to you the moment you were conceived in My Grace. No one and nothing can supplant the value I have bestowed upon you and in you. The world at this time and this place is more valuable because you are alive. Your body is the temple of My Spirit. Treat your body with kindness and respect and you will find healthy joy.

When life confronts you with earthly choices that are not good for you, remember to lift your chin and seek Me. I have given you the will and the power to overcome any temptation. Believe in My strength as I believe in yours. Listen well to My voice and My whispers, not the sirens of this earth. I tell you, My child, aim high, and

I will help you soar higher. From the moment you were born, I have charged you with great commands. Do you hear them? Do you obey them? Follow your inner spirit and set your goals on Me. I will lead you toward earthly success and, more importantly, eternal reward. You are human, yet I am divine. Trust in Me, and I will give you the strength you need to change your life from the inside out. No matter what this world brings you, remember you are invaluably valuable. I am the Fire but you are My flame. Ignite your inner light for the entire world to see. The greater My Spirit shines in you and through you, the more you illuminate dark paths for others. Let not this world give you direction, but rather, you direct the world.

Navigate your way through Me, and I will guide you on the right path, the one chosen uniquely for you. I will never steer you down the wrong path, and I will never forsake you. Lift your feet and run for Me. Let me be your Guide, and I will gently aid you in self-control and healthy choices. When you choose Me, you choose Love. I am always with you, even when you feel alone and afraid and desperate. Remember, I am your Ultimate Pacer and the only Celebrity Trainer you will ever need. In My arms, you will always find rest, for you are forever wrapped and embraced in My Unconditional Love.

Molly Wade – *Madbury, NH*

get in the word

1 Samuel 16:7

But the Lord said to Samuel, "Do not look at his appearance or at his physical stature, because I have refused him. For the Lord does not see as man sees; for man looks at the outward appearance, but the Lord looks at the heart."

Isaiah 64:8

But now, O Lord,
You are our Father;
We are the clay, and You our potter;
And all we are the work of Your hand.

1 Corinthians 6:19

Or do you not know that your body is the temple of the Holy Spirit who is in you, whom you have from God, and you are not your own?

scripture memorization

Write out the scripture(s) in the space below and recite them ten times.

something to ponder

DOES SOCIETY'S messages about your body or weight inhibit you from being your true self?

DO YOU make time to listen to God? His voice is not always as loud as those around us. Can you hear Him through the earthly noise and static? What is He saying?

EACH OF us has an inner spark. We need to fan our flames in order to set the world on fire for Him. How can you share your light with others?

running observations by dean

Connect Action with Goals

GOALS ARE ESSENTIAL TO SUCCESS IN all that we do, yet we don't always take time to develop those goals. If you are going from day to day with no real focus on a running goal, stop what you are doing and take some time to decide what you want to accomplish. Whether your goal is to finish a half marathon or to run a 10K faster than you have ever run one before, having the goal crystal clear in front of you will improve your chances of success. If you haven't taken time to find that goal, do it now.

Today, I have a goal for a race that is over six months away. I know what I want to accomplish, and I will think about that goal nearly every day, relentlessly pursuing it. I won't obsess over it or make it the center of my everyday life, but I know it and will think about it every time I go out to run. Goals require action. If I don't put action behind the thoughts that I have about my goal, I won't get there. I can want to go to New York and even pick my route on a map, but until I begin the process of packing, fueling the car, making the turns as I drive, checking the traffic around me, stopping to refuel my car and my body, etc., I will never make it. There are a lot of things to do (action) to complete the trip. What if I skip a step, like eating on the way? I might get there, but I probably won't enjoy myself very much once I do because I'll be cranky!

The point is that you have to pursue your goals daily, and running is no different from other endeavors. There are a lot of turns to make, places to stop, and delays because of road construction along the way, but remaining in motion and moving towards the goal, in one way or another, is important. I have heard many regrets on race day where someone didn't do all the work needed to make the race all it could be. You do not want to be that person. Of course, there will be adjustments along the way. There will be days when something comes up, and you can't execute the plan the way you want to, but don't let it stop you from executing a plan.

When it is tough to go out and run, think about your goal even more intensely. Feel the exhilaration of success as you imagine yourself accomplishing your goal. Now, it's time to do something to get there. What step do you have to take today? Don't think about how hard that step is, think about what's at the top waiting for you at the end of all those steps.

James 1:2-4 reads, "My brethren, count it all joy when you fall into various trials, knowing that the testing of your faith produces patience. But let patience have its perfect work, that you may be perfect and complete, lacking nothing." Just like trying to get through a tough running day, God allows us to face tough obstacles in life. Those trials make us stronger and move us toward our goal of being more like Christ. We will never be the fastest runners in the world, but we can be faster when we run through the tough days. When we completely trust Him in those times of trials, He tells us we will lack nothing, because He will make us more complete. Wow.

- *Make sure you have gone through the process of setting a goal that you can focus on.*
- *Relentlessly pursue your goal with action, not just words or thoughts.*
- *Facing the valleys in life is tough, but God tells us that He will make us stronger when we rely on Him and keep moving through them.*

from the inside out

"FROM THE INSIDE OUT" SOMETIMES LIFE snaps in half. Boom. The life you once knew cracks; your "normal" disappears. That's what happened to me. At 35 years old, my world ended. Running saved my life. To be precise, running for God saved my life.

Bad things aren't supposed to happen to good people. At least, that's what I thought. Growing up a good Catholic girl, I always did the right things. I was a good daughter, a good sister, a good friend, and a good student. I got married and became a good wife and, shortly afterwards, I became a good mother. Being "good" was all I knew how to be. It came naturally to me, it was how I was raised to be, it was my instinctual response, but then, my goodness intersected with badness. My husband surrendered to the habits of a full-fledged alcoholic. He drank at home, and he drank away from home. His anger issues went from disruptive and uncomfortable to abusive and unmanageable, and one day, his behavior finally crossed the threshold of miserably tolerable to absolutely intolerable. I crumbled.

Actually, I crumpled. I fell to the floor and screamed at God. I shook my fist at heaven and demanded a do-over. Here I was, a young mother with four small children, and I had been pushed head first into a cataclysmic disturbance of thunder, lightning and hurricane winds, all at once. I found myself at the center of the perfect storm, and I had no idea how to navigate my way through it. Divorce? Suicide? Accept perpetual torture? All entered my mind, all seemed unsatisfactory options. I began to run. I ran and cried and cried and ran. While I ran, I screamed. I screamed at God, at the Universe, at Goodness, at Time (especially at time). There was so much of it left. I was just 35 years old and there seemingly was so much time left before God might consider providing me the reprieve of death. To a heart filled with grief, death seems like a relief, a reward, and a respite.

I ran more, and while I ran, I talked at God, not with Him. My conversations with God went something like this: I prayed for the end of the world, I prayed for the rapture, I prayed for the apocalypse. I wept, pleaded, begged, borrowed, negotiated and bribed. I prayed for mercy, for guidance, for comfort, for death, for healing. I wasn't Jesus. I couldn't be expected to carry this impossibly heavy cross through life. My voice was loud. God's voice was quiet. My voice quivered. His was steady. His unwavering and outstretched hand made me-mad. I wanted Him to take justice out on those who had hurt me. Forgiveness was not an option I was seeking. Even an "eye for an eye" didn't seem a fair enough punishment. So, I ran harder. When it hurt, I ran further. Maybe redemptive suffering would erase the pain of my husband's sins. Maybe God would give me His grace.

Was God even there? Turns out, He was. My husband recognized that he had reached rock bottom and stopped drinking. He sought help and entered a recovery program. It didn't fix my brokenness, but it helped. I kept running. Over time, my running feet took me through many paths. I ran on asphalt. I ran through woods.

I ran when the sun rose, I ran when the sun set. I ran and ran and ran. The tears dried, the anxiety lessened, the aching dulled, and the hatred waned. Forgiveness seeped into my heart where once only anger and bitterness resided. Endurance and perseverance became my allies; strength and fortitude became my one-word mantras. "I can do this," I muttered when my body swore differently. I ran when my feet blistered, when my knees ached and when my legs throbbed. The throbbing in my body helped numb the throbbing in my heart. Love was lost, but life was not. My newly realized virtues emboldened me to begin new ministries at church: first one, then two, then three. I used my pain and my suffering to comfort others. Compassion became my first outburst. Running helped me realize that although my "normal" would never be the same, I (the person I knew myself to be) was essentially the same - whole, complete, and yes, good.

Although my husband, society, culture, and the world tried to break me (and admittedly, they did temporarily break me) they did not destroy me. Nothing and no one can do that with God by my side. Today, I don't suffer from intense hurt. The scars will last forever, but scars aren't altogether bad things. They serve as reminders of what was, what to avoid, and the blessings of healing. Running brings me clarity, comfort, and peace. Most of the time I run alone, sometimes I run with my now sober husband, always I run with God. He is my truest running partner, my singular pacer, and my celebrity trainer. Without Him, running would only mean moving my feet in a general direction. With Him, each step has meaning, focus, intention, and will. So, whatever life brings me, I lift my feet and I run for God. He is my starting line and my finish line; He high fives me at every mile marker. And he cheers for me from the inside out. I just know it.

Molly Wade – *Madbury, NH*

get in the word

Philippians 4:13

I can do all things through Christ who strengthens me.

Matthew 5:38

You have heard that it was said, 'An eye for an eye and a tooth for a tooth.'

Matthew 6:14-15

For if you forgive men their trespasses, your heavenly Father will also forgive you. But if you do not forgive men their trespasses, neither will your Father forgive your trespasses.

scripture memorization

Write out the scripture(s) in the space below and recite them ten times.

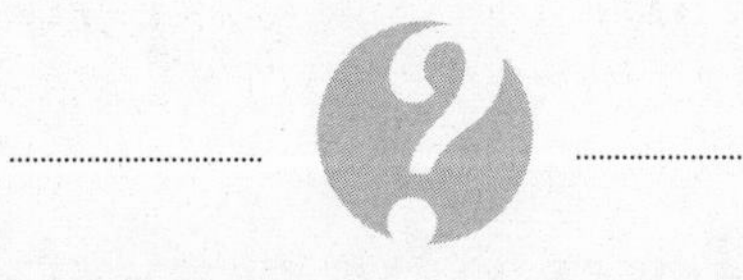

something to ponder

WHAT CROSSES do you carry that inhibit you to run freely?

How can "letting go and letting God" allow you to run faster, farther, and freely throughout life?

DO YOU place your trust in and evaluate your self-worth by the things of this world or the things born of God? How do they differ? Which is more reliable?

---

running observations by dean

Running the Tangents

THE EASIEST WAY FOR MOST RUNNERS to pick up a few seconds on the race course is to run the tangents. No, a tangent isn't some new training technique. If you paid attention in geometry class, you may remember what a tangent is. If you were not a math geek, a tangent is a line that touches a curve but does not cross the line of the curve. If you run around a track, it may be easier to explain this way:

Running in lane two would cause you to run longer than someone in lane one. The inside of lane one is the shortest possible route around a track and running the tangents on a race course means running the shortest possible route.

Picture a course where you have to make a right turn, run one block and then make a left turn. Most runners will run along one side of the road and then cut over at the last second. The shortest possible route would take you diagonally across the street to form a straight line from one turn to the next. The same thing applies to running on a curved road. Many runners will stay on one side of the road, but that is not usually the shortest possible route. Running from the inside of one curve to the inside of the next curve will be significantly shorter.

Is it cheating to cross the road? Actually, by following the shortest possible route, you are following the same route that is measured when the course was certified (if it is a certified course). Often, when I am talking to runners after a race, the discussion will get to the length of the course. Inevitably, someone will point to their GPS watch and say, "The course was too long. I got 6.34 miles." Since it is almost impossible to run a perfect line throughout an entire race, we will all run a little farther than the measured length. If your GPS watch tells you that you ran exactly the race distance, chances are good that either your watch did not measure accurately, or the course is a little short.

When a course is certified, there are very strict procedures that include calibration of equipment and multiple measurements to ensure accuracy. The procedures are designed to produce a course that is never too short. A great course measurer will be accurate to within inches. That's why it is not only okay to take the shortest possible route, but it is the right thing to do.

A couple of words of caution: 1) Trying to follow the shortest possible route in a large race with thousands of participants is difficult. It is not advisable to push through crowds trying to get to the next corner in the shortest line. It would be rude and it may not end pretty. 2) Many courses are open to traffic. Safety always comes first. Do not try to follow the shortest possible route when your safety is at stake!

There is no variability in the route to Heaven. Jesus said in Matthew 7:13-14, "Enter by the narrow gate; for wide is the gate and broad is the way that leads to destruction, and there are many who go in by it. Because narrow is the gate and difficult is the way which leads to life, and there are few who find it." Although there may be many paths to take in service to our Lord, there is only one way to get to Heaven. Believe in what He did for us on the cross, submit to Him and you will find the narrow gate.

- *Running the tangents on the race course ensures the shortest possible run, resulting in the fastest possible time.*
- *Courses are measured to make sure you run at least the race distance.*
- *There is one way to Heaven.*

____

____

____

running faster with God

APRIL 15, 2013, WAS A DAY I will not forget, even though I was not in my birthplace, Boston, Massachusetts. Even though I live in the South, New England is where I grew up and will always consider my home. This particular day started my running life.

I had run track in school, but when I neared the age of 50, running was not something I ever thought I would do. I vowed I would run races the next year honoring my city. I started training for a half marathon. Most people would have started with a 5k, but I was going for what I felt was the GOLD. As I trained, I would listen to music and run. Unfortunately, my head still thought I was 17, but my body and legs were saying "nope you're 50". My music contained the typical upbeat list, but when I would tire, it didn't help much. I asked God to keep me going for 5 more minutes to give my legs a little extra go. One day, I changed my music to Christian Contemporary and without missing a beat, my time got faster, and my legs felt stronger to go that extra mile.

Before I knew it, my half marathon arrived, and my head was full of doubt. I was scared to death, but I knew God was with me and would give me everything I needed. When the race began, my inspirational music played, and I ran. I did not run the entire race, but I was okay with it. When I got tired, God's words filled my ears.

I had only a mile to go, and my eyes filled with tears. I was really going to make it. I started thanking God for allowing me to complete my race. That last mile was full of thankfulness. When I crossed the finish line, I knew that "with God" all things are possible.

At 50 years old, I finished my first half marathon on February 2014. Since that day, I have completed another half marathon, a 10K and a 5K, with a goal to complete two more half marathons and a few more 5Ks before the year's end. I may have started running because of what happened on April 15, 2013, but if it weren't for that day, I wouldn't have started and continued to run for Him.

Noreen Kent – *Indian Land, SC*

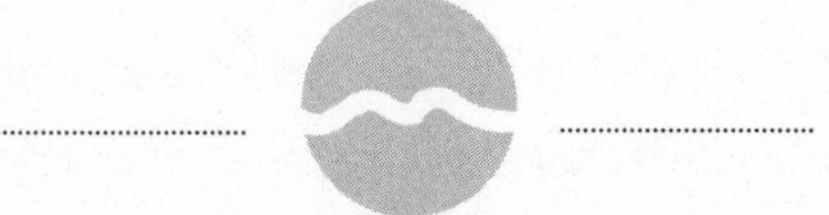

get in the word

2 Corinthians 12:9-10

And He said to me, "My grace is sufficient for you, for my strength is made perfect in weakness." Therefore most gladly I will rather boast in my infirmities, that the power of Christ may rest upon me. Therefore I take pleasure in infirmities, in reproaches, in needs, in persecutions, in distresses, for Christ's sake. For when I am weak, then I am strong.

Mark 10:27

But Jesus looked at them and said, "With men it is impossible, but not with God; for with God all things are possible."

Isaiah 40:31

But those who wait on the Lord shall renew their strength; they shall mount up with wings like eagles, they shall run and not be weary, they shall walk and not faint.

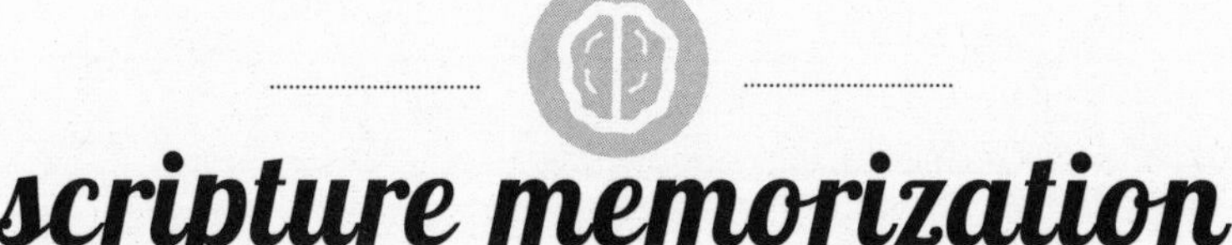

scripture memorization

Write out the scripture(s) in the space below and recite them ten times.

something to ponder

CAN WE overcome anything with God? Is there anything we cannot accomplish with His help?

DO WE have to be perfect?

DO YOU trust God?

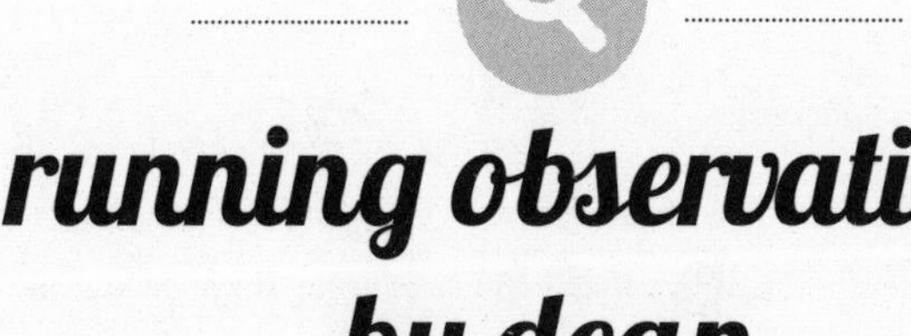

running observations by dean

Post Run Weight Gain Mistakes

YOU RUN ALMOST EVERY DAY AND still have more weight hanging on your frame than you want. There are several reasons why it may be a problem for you, and some of them may be caused by good intentions. What do you do immediately following a run? If you have done any research on the subject, you know that a post run dose of protein with some carbohydrates will help your muscles begin the rebuilding process more quickly. In fact, you will find advocates for drinking chocolate milk after a run for the protein boost. While it's true that it will help, if you drink twice as much as prescribed, you can do more harm than good. I don't know about you, but it's hard for me to stop drinking chocolate milk once I get started! It is important, however, to eat a snack after running. Just be careful what it is and how much you consume.

Another way you can short circuit yourself is to reward yourself too much. If you have a difficult time motivating yourself to run, you may find yourself setting rewards for when you reach milestones. It's a great tool, but be careful. If you are rewarding yourself with junk food, you may be partially or completely negating the benefits of the run. Remember, calories burned should be more than calories consumed.

Drinking sports drinks is another way to sabotage your efforts. While they have their place during long workouts, the sugar in most sports drinks will turn to fat once processed by your body. If you're not running for at least an hour, the electrolytes in these drinks are unnecessary anyway. Drink water instead, or find a healthier alternative.

The importance of consistent exercise cannot be overstated. If you run every day this week but none next week, it is not as good as running three or four days both weeks. If you use the fact that you are tired or sore to not run today, it can turn into two days and then three, etc. Scheduling your runs ahead of time is critical to weight loss success. You should always know when your next run will be. If you don't have a weekly plan for your runs, make a habit of planning your next run as soon as you complete today's run. Do your absolute best to maintain your commitment to your workouts. While there are certainly times when things come up that require you to change your plans, make sure the reason is really important enough to warrant giving up a run.

Finally, don't skip your post run stretch or cross training exercises that make you stronger. If you are injured because you neglected these things, you may pay the price in weight gain.

Daily prayer and Bible study get tough when life is happening around us. If we rely on trying to fit God into our daily plans, we will likely be just as successful with it as we are when we don't plan our runs. Psalms 46:1 reads, "God is our refuge and strength, a very present help in trouble." It's important to schedule your time with God to gain that strength. He should receive priority over everything else we do. When we plan to run and then execute the plan, we feel better physically. When we plan our time with God and then execute, we feel better spiritually.

- *You may be inadvertently sabotaging your effort to lose weight.*
- *Be smart about the way you plan your runs and what you do after each run.*
- *Daily time with God makes us stronger spiritually.*

Endure the Race

I'VE BEEN BLESSED ENOUGH TO RUN the race a few times. The first time I signed up for a 5k, I placed myself into the unknown. I thought, "How hard can it be to move or try to pass someone rapidly or even just complete a 3.1 mile run just for fun?" Well, the question then became, "When does running get easier?" Some days during training, I wanted to pull my hair out and punch the wall, but eventually, I found out that running was helping me get through other pains and frustrations. I find IT difficult to explain what drives me to run, but running has changed my life. I never thought I had what it takes to be a "runner" until I accepted the challenge to follow the right habits to reach the goal-the finish line.

Running is not only a great form of exercise, but also running gives me a feeling of strength and freedom. Every time I run, I believe there is a finish line, and to get there, I must keep running, knowing that every step brings me closer. I'm currently training for my 6th race, and it is still a challenge. Sometimes, it feels like it is the ultimate test of physical endurance, but every time I run, I'm learning to hang in there, I'm learning to be determined, and I'm challenging myself all over again. I must finish!

Push yourself through the pain! Don't stop running! Don't stop running just because you are exhausted or have a cramp in your side. Keep going! Somehow, at the end of the race, the pain will be worth the prize. We push beyond the pain and look ahead to the finish line. We hold on! We trust! We endure! Run the race with endurance!
Hebrews 12:1

Frances Agosto – *Orlando, FL*

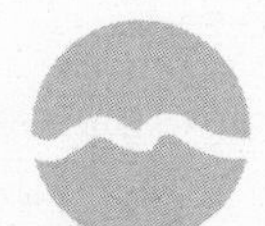

get in the word

Hebrews 12:1
Therefore we also, since we are surrounded by so great a cloud of witnesses, let us lay aside every weight, and the sin which so easily ensnares us, and let us run with endurance the race that is set before us,

Hebrews 12:2
Looking unto Jesus, the author and finisher of our faith, who for the joy that was set before Him endured the cross, despising the shame,

and has sat down at the right hand of the throne of God.

scripture memorization

Write out the scripture(s) in the space below and recite them ten times.

____

____

____

____

____

something to ponder

WHAT IS your focus while on the race?

LIST AND rank the significance of anything that is or might hinder you from enduring the race?

____

____

____

____

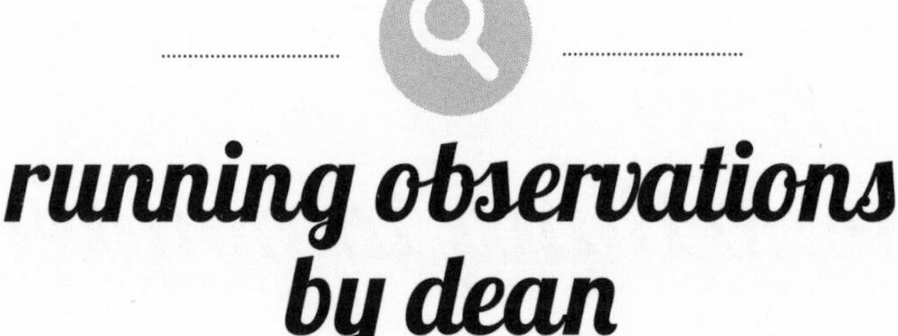

Hills on Purpose

I KNOW A FEW PEOPLE WHO tell me they like to run hills. I don't know if they are fibbing to me or if they really do like to run hills. Either way, they are in the minority because our collective feeling about hills ranges from, "they're a nuisance" to "I'd rather have a root canal than run up one more hill." However, there are many reasons to run hills, even seek them out and embrace them. Running hills can make you faster and less injury prone. They can increase power, endurance, speed, and can help you run with better form. In short, running hills is a no-brainer if you want to be a better runner. Do you feel better about hills yet?

When you run uphill, your effort level has to increase to keep the same pace. You breathe much harder with the intensification of effort. This stresses your aerobic system, increasing your ability to process oxygen which improves overall endurance. Once you get to a point where you cannot continue that effort, you begin to use more oxygen than you are taking in, leading to stress on your anaerobic system and pushing your anaerobic threshold higher. Both of these lead to being able to maintain a faster pace with less effort for your easy runs, which, in turn, allows you to run faster races. Do you feel better about hills yet?

When you run uphill, you must lift your knees higher because of the required lift to get to higher ground. In addition, using your arms helps to create more lift, so you automatically increase the use of your arms. Presto, you are running with better form. If you do it enough, this more efficient form of running will transfer to your running on flat ground. When running economy increases, you get faster. Do you feel better about hills yet?

The increased effort combined with the decreased impact of running uphill leads to stronger muscles and more power. What follows is insulation from injury. Anyone want to be injury free?

If you are going to begin running hills, there are a few things you need to know before getting started. First, only begin intentional hill work once you have worked your way up to at least fifteen miles per week. If you are a beginner, make sure you have a sufficient base before your first hill workout. Second, make sure you warm up and cool down before subjecting your body to the increased stress that hills will provide. Stretch well, too. Third, start slowly by only running hill workouts once every two or three weeks. It will take time to recover from the effort.

Once you have decided to run hills on purpose, you will have to decide how to do it. You can choose to run hill repeats where you run up a hill and walk or jog back down only to turn around and do it again. If you are new to hill training, start with only four to six repetitions to see what effect it will have on your body. Or, you can run hilly routes and focus your effort particularly on running hard up the hills. Once again, take it easy on the downhills and flat sections if you are new to powering up hills.

Finally, if you live in an area where there are no hills, you have to be creative. You can find a bridge or a parking garage to use for incline. If that is not possible, there's always the treadmill. Raise the incline on the treadmill to 5% then 8% and run for a minute or two at a time. It's not as fun, but it is effective.

I know people who prefer to read and study from the New Testament, forsaking the wordy and seemingly less interesting Old Testament. Sure the New Covenant of the New Testament is the lynchpin of our faith, but there is so much depth in the Old Testament. The prophecies alone are fascinating to study, but add the incredible stories that have so much relevance to today and it is a treasure trove of faith building knowledge. In addition, Psalms and Proverbs are incredibly inspirational. There is a reason why God preserved the Bible in its entirety for so many years. It's a good idea for us to make use of everything between the covers.

- *Very few people will admit to liking hills.*

- *Running hills will make you faster and less injury prone.*

- *There is not an irrelevant word in the Bible.*

sticky notes

45
Week

just do it

PRAISE THE LORD! FOR THE FIRST time ever - I RAN 3 MILES FOR GOD AND WITH GOD WITHOUT STOPPING! I just decided to forget the time and JUST DO IT FOR THE GLORY OF THE LORD!

I had slacked on the diet and the exercise during a difficult season of my life. I changed my route a little and the breeze was nice. I had several red bird sightings, which are significantly meaningful to me with my dad passing in February. I have seen a red bird almost every day since he passed. The second round, I saw a bird flying circles over my house which reminded me of the words of Psalm 139:5, “Behind and before you encircle me and rest your hand upon me.”

I had never run over two miles before. As my legs felt the distance, I told myself I would not stop until I got the victory, so I kept on running. As I neared the last mile, there was a bird waiting for me on top of a stop sign as if it were watching me race to the finish line. On the last stretch to the third mile, I look up to see a flock of birds flying in my same direction as if they were racing against me. As I neared the finish line, the breeze picked up and the leaves rustled in the wind as if they were cheering for me. Leaves fell from the trees above me as if they were confetti being dropped from above as I broke through the finish line. Then my phone app came on and announced my time as I completed 3 miles in a time better than ever before.

I am glad no one was watching as I raised my arms in victory after having finished the 3-mile race I thought I would never complete. I had won and I didn't stop. I ran all the way home with a huge smile of victory covering my face. It spoke volumes to my heart and soul during this difficult time in my life. My job seemed insecure and unfulfilling. My dad passed away, and my mom had a near-death experience. My child was very sick. Problems come at me right and left, but I am determined to keep running until victorious, as I did today in my Run for God. The words of the song that was playing rang so true in my heart..."There's no struggle you can't face... Our God His love will never fail.... Strong through every storm..."

Christy Hardy – *Northport, AL*

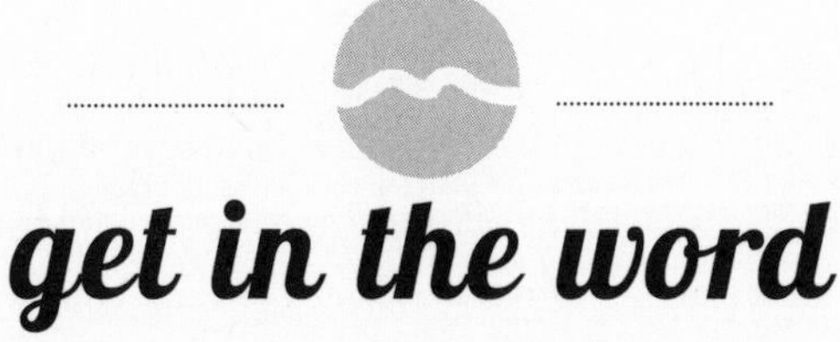

Psalm 139:5

You have hedged me behind and before, and laid Your hand upon me.

Psalm 18:2
The Lord is my rock and my fortress and my deliverer; my God, my strength, in whom I will trust; my shield and the horn of my salvation, my stronghold.

1 Corinthians 15:57
But thanks be to God, who gives us the victory through our Lord Jesus Christ.

scripture memorization

Write out the scripture(s) in the space below and recite them ten times.

something to ponder

HOW WOULD an awareness of God's presence encircling you change what you do and say today?

HAS THERE been a time in your life when Christ was your strong tower?

____

____

____

____

OVER WHAT has Christ given you victory?

____

____

____

____

running observations by dean

Half Marathon Madness

SURVEY RESULTS RELEASED IN MAY OF 2015 by Running USA reported that, for the first time ever, there were over two million finishers in all Half Marathons in 2014. That number was up over ten percent from the previous year. The average age was 37, with a 61 percent to 39 percent female to male ratio. Breaking down the age further, 4 percent were under 20 years old, 54 percent were 20 – 39 and 42 percent were over 40.

What does all that mean? I think it's a great statement about our sport! Whether you are a new runner who has never thought about attempting a half marathon, or you have completed dozens of them, this is good news for all of us.

For the new runner who has never conquered the distance, this report indicates that you can do it because so many others have done it! There's a reason why the average time to complete a half marathon increases every year; many of the newcomers are those who have had doubts about just how large a mountain they could scale prior to the completion of their first half (an abbreviation the veterans like to use). More and more people are realizing that they can do more than they ever thought possible, and so can you. How about you? Are you ready to burn even more calories? Are you ready to put a little more structure into your training? Are you ready to expand the number of runners you know by meeting more people? Are you ready for the lifetime of bragging rights that come with crossing that finish line? What are you waiting for?

Have you already run ten half marathons? This news is good for you too. The more people who participate in them, the more opportunities there will be to run them as organizers develop more races. There were over 400 half marathons with over 1,000 participants in 2014. There are many to choose from and, if the trend continues, there will be many more to choose from in the future. If you are a front-of-the-pack runner, never forget that it is the average-paced runner who makes the race possible.

I have a couple of negative observations about half marathons, too. Ten mile races are getting as scarce as hen's teeth. Many race organizers have opted to change their ten mile races to the more appealing half marathon distance. It's not a big deal, but us older folks remember when there were many ten milers to choose from. And, finally, my only real issue with the half marathon is this: Can't we change the name? Do you think the term says, "I'm only half as good as a marathoner?" Or, does the fact that the word "marathon" is most of the title tell you that it is almost a marathon? I don't know which way to go, and that's the problem!

Seriously, a half marathon is a great accomplishment. If you haven't tried to tackle the distance yet, consider taking it on in the future. It's a 1-2-3 process: 1) Sign up for a race. 2) Train for a race. 3) Race the race! It's that easy! Okay, there are some details to tackle in between, but you're up to it!

Jesus said in Matthew 17:20, "for assuredly, I say to you, if you have faith as a mustard seed, you will say to this mountain, 'Move from here to there,' and it will move; and nothing will be impossible for you." Jesus is telling the disciples that they are selling themselves short. They don't realize the power that faith will provide them. If you are selling yourself short, thinking you can't do something, a little faith combined with hard work can get you there. Even better, God will be with you every step of the way!

- *There are more half marathon finishers today than ever before because more people realize they can do it.*

- *Whether you are a new runner or a seasoned veteran, there are reasons to celebrate the explosion of the half marathon.*

- *Jesus tells us that we can conquer more than we think we can if we will only have faith.*

sticky notes

stepping out

I CAN'T EVEN BEGIN TO ATTEMPT to understand the mystery of God. He has plans for me, knows my needs before I know them, and has all of the answers before I even ask. Isaiah 55:8 says, "For my thoughts are not your thoughts, neither are your ways my ways," declares the Lord." According to this verse, I don't even think that I could come anywhere near to understanding the "whys" and "whats" of the Lord's plans for me.

After an emotionally and mentally tough weekend, I have learned one thing, which is to trust Him wholly and completely. In my current situation, I am desperately clinging to Him and having a complete blind faith because I am stepping out on a new adventure that is a little scary for me. This isn't scary because it's new; it's scary because there are others involved. Others who have emotions and thoughts and my decision could affect them. For three days, I prayed and scoured scripture before I made a decision. There were two verses that stood out and gave me peace and reassurance: Jeremiah 29:11 and Psalm 119:32.

One of my fears was that I could not run harder and longer. In the past few days, I have pushed myself to run harder than I have before and the same thoughts kept rolling through my mind, "Take me deeper than my feet could ever wander and my faith will be made stronger." These lyrics are from a beautiful worship song "Oceans" by Hillsong United. I trusted that God would give me the strength to push myself harder during my run, and in that small, menial part of my life, it caused me to trust Him in bigger things. When I finished my run, I realized if God could give me enough strength to get over a tiny fear of running harder, why wouldn't He give me the strength to begin something new in my life? The answer is obvious. He will give me the strength to do this, and He'll be there every step of the way guiding me and leading me. I trusted that God would take me places I would never think to go, and in this, my faith would increase because I would have no other choice but to have faith and to trust.

Ashley Marshall – Garland, TX

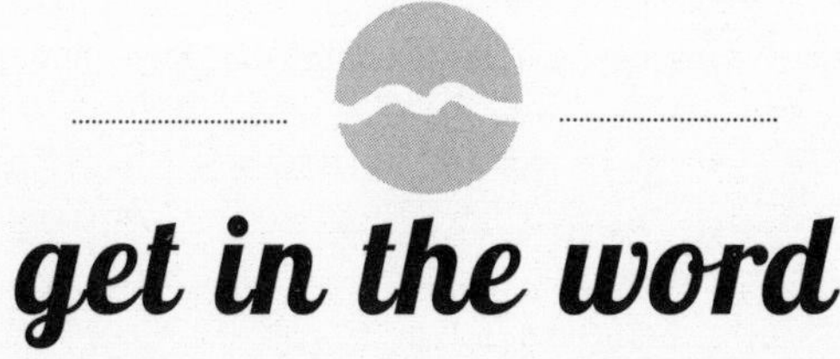

Isaiah 55:8

"For My thoughts are not your thoughts, nor are your ways My ways," says the Lord.

Jeremiah 29:11

For I know the thoughts that I think toward you, says the Lord, thoughts of peace and not of evil, to give you a future and a hope.

Psalm 119:32

I will run the course of Your commandments, for You shall enlarge my heart.

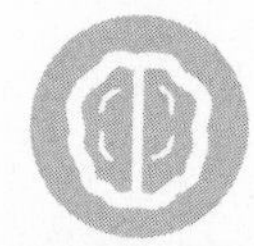

scripture memorization

Write out the scripture(s) in the space below and recite them ten times.

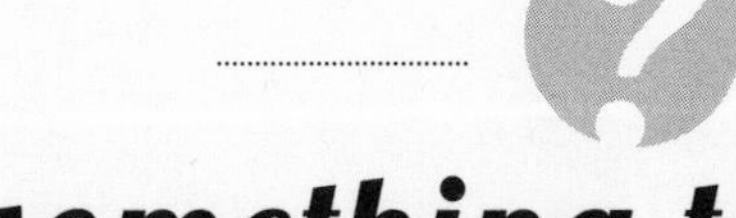

something to ponder

WHAT WOULD it take to step out and push yourself out of your comfort zone?

WHERE DO you find your strength to push through and finish a tough run?

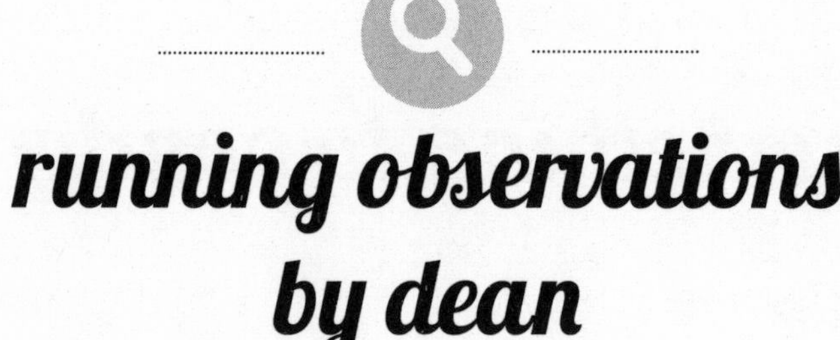

Treadmill Running

I'M SURE THERE ARE PEOPLE WHO enjoy running on a treadmill, but I don't know any of them. When we spend so much time outside, enjoying the scenery while we traverse country roads or city streets, it's tough to go inside and run in one place. If you live in a place where the weather is so extreme you cannot run outside, you either have to take time off, or face the treadmill. If you take too much time off, it becomes difficult to get started again. You expose your body to higher injury risk each time you have to start over, making the treadmill more attractive. Not to mention, the sheer difficulty of beginning again can be daunting!

Fortunately, there are things you can do with a treadmill to make it less boring due to the lack of scenery change. Many people hop on the treadmill, find a comfortable setting and just run, perhaps changing speeds to allow for a warm up and cool down. Here are some things you can do to mix it up:

Change something every quarter or half mile. Change the incline or your speed. If you know the terrain of an upcoming race, you can use the incline on the treadmill to simulate the hills on the race course. If you speed the belt up for a minute or two, you'll find it easier to return to the slower pace. Changing the settings will help keep you engaged in something other than watching the time go by.

Check your form. Monitor your form every half mile, making sure that your arms are swinging parallel to each other and are at a ninety degree angle. Don't slouch, push your hips forward, and relax your shoulders. Practice keeping your form sharp on inclines, as well. Count your strides and ensure that your cadence is where it should be. Count how many times your right foot hits the treadmill for one minute. It should be between 83 and 93.

Entertain yourself. This one is obvious, but watching television or listening to music, a podcast, or a book are great ways to keep your mind occupied for those long treadmill miles. I watched an entire series while riding my bike on a trainer preparing for a triathlon.

Do an interval workout. Warm up for a mile or two then run hard for a mile. Back your speed down to something very easy for a half-mile, and go back to running hard again. You can vary the distances of the hard runs and easy runs. Try different combinations, or make it part of your overall training plan.

Pray every mile. Write down some people for whom you want to pray, and pray for one each mile on the treadmill. You don't want to substitute this time for quiet time with Him, but it can be a great supplement.

Stay positive. This sounds too easy to actually work, but it does. Don't go into a treadmill session with dread. Have a positive attitude, knowing that you are better preparing yourself for the good weather to come.

Two separate runs. If it's still too much, break your run into two sessions, running the first in the morning and the second in the evening. It's not as good as one run, but it's very close.

Hopefully, you don't have to run on the treadmill every day, but there are areas of the country where running outside is difficult for extended periods of time. If you are one who must use the treadmill for more than a few weeks, be careful when you go back outside. Move your shorter runs outside first and get your body used to the difference.

There are days when it is more difficult than others, but the treadmill doesn't have to be a dreadful experience. Sometimes Bible study can be difficult, too. We get so busy with life that we have to cut things out of our day because we can't get to them all. Often, our daily time in God's word suffers because we are busy, but also because we sometimes look at it like we see the treadmill. But, Bible study doesn't have to be restricted to opening to a page and simply reading. We can study topics or dive deeply into a particular book, or we can dwell on one verse for a week. When we take the time to study His word, it makes the rest of the day so much better. When we have to put something aside, we need to make sure that it is something other than our time with Him. 2Timothy 3:16-17 says, "All Scripture is given by inspiration of God, and is profitable for doctrine, for reproof, for correction, for instruction in righteousness, that the man of God may be complete, thoroughly equipped for every good work." Well, that explains it!

- *Running on a treadmill is not the best way to experience running, but there are things you can do to make is less monotonous.*

- *Try changing speeds or the incline while you run to keep your mind occupied. If that doesn't work, try television or music.*

- *Some of us don't like to read anything, and it makes Bible study difficult, but there are things you can do during Bible study to make it easier and more fulfilling.*

47
Week

my first 5k

WHEN I BEGAN THE COUCH TO 5K program, I was not planning on running my first 5K four weeks later. The last time I had run was in junior high, and I was a sprinter. To be perfectly honest, I really had no desire to run until a few months ago. A new challenge to my workout was what I was seeking. I kept praying to find the right fit for me, and God was leading me to running.

At first, I was not very receptive to the idea of running. God and I had some interesting conversations on the matter, and I kept saying, "God, this is not what I had in mind, can't you come up with something else?" Obviously, God won. I knew I had to trust God to take me on this journey. I had yet to realize that running would not just help transform me physically, but mentally, emotionally and spiritually. After consulting with my running friends for advice, I was told to go to The Starting Block for a gait analysis, so I would have the proper shoes to avoid injury. Well, I got the shoes and was told about a Couch to 5K eight-week program that was going to start and was encouraged to join. With nervous hesitation, I did. The first night of the Couch to 5K program, I was nervous and excited. Progress was made each week, and as I saw this progression, my confidence began to increase. The fourth week was upon me, and I had a choice to make: meet with the group at our regular time or take the opportunity to run a 5K our coach was assisting with in Branson. My husband and I went to Branson for our first 5K run; a decision that impacted me more than I ever would have imagined.

Here it was—the day of the Freedom Run of the Ozarks. I did not sleep well, had butterflies in my stomach, and kept waking up every two hours. Nervous, obviously, but more importantly, I was excited and happy that I was following through on something I had started with God and had my husband by my side. I had not set any goals other than to finish and enjoy the run. The whistle had blown, and we had begun to run. Here I was, my husband standing in front of me, my coach standing beside me, and the Holy Spirit within me, all encouraging me with each step I took. My pace was good and I felt strong. I enjoyed the company and the beautiful scenery God provided all around me. Before I knew it, I was halfway done.

Then, I saw it—the finish line. I began to run faster. I felt the tears in my eyes. I was surprised by the emotion that I felt, but I could not let it get to me before I had crossed that line. A hug from my husband and then my coach was the best way to end the run and then the tears of joy flooded me. Now, I am blessed to coach the group that got me started. All the glory goes to God.

Kesta Smith – *Nixa, AL*

get in the word

Philippians 4:13
I can do all things through Christ who strengthens me.

Psalm 139:13-14
For You formed my inward parts; You covered me in my mother's womb. I will praise You, for I am fearfully and wonderfully made; Marvelous are Your works, And that my soul knows very well.

Joshua 1:9

Have I not commanded you? Be strong and of good courage; do not be afraid, nor be dismayed, for the Lord your God is with you wherever you go.

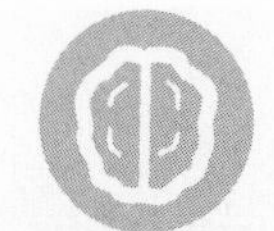

scripture memorization

Write out the scripture(s) in the space below and recite them ten times.

____

____

____

____

something to ponder

WHY DO we let fear control us? In Joshua 1:9, God commands us to be courageous.

____

____

ISN'T IT important to take care of the body God gave us? If we don't we cannot tell the world about Jesus.

____

____

____

____

WHY DO we stay in our comfort zone? Being comfortable can limit our growth in our faith.

____

____

____

running observations by dean

Girly Girl Runners

IN GENERAL, MANY PEOPLE DO NOT list sports as highly feminine. I'm not saying that it's right or wrong to see it that way, only making a general observation. When we look at participation rates in sports, the female percentage is usually a fraction of the male participation. Of course, there are exceptions, and running is one of them. It is a sport for everyone, even girly girls! I know a lot of female runners who really don't care much for sports in general but love running. It is the time when they don't care about the hair and makeup, even in public. Somehow, it is okay to sweat when you're running, even if it is unacceptable nearly any other time.

There are several reasons why I think running has this positive standing with these ladies. For starters, running is a great way to stay slim, toned and healthy. It is totally worth the effort because the rewards are substantial. Fitting into smaller clothing is certainly right up the girly-girl alley! In addition, having the ability to remain more active throughout the day just helps to get more done.

Saturday mornings are completely different socially! Meeting up with friends and like-minded people gives them an additional reason to show up on race morning. The social interaction is something everyone looks forward to, and it is no different for this segment of the running world. According to studies, women use an average of 20,000 words a day. Saturday morning group runs and races provide a platform to use a bunch of them up early!

The clothing is cool! Running has its own fashion and the choices are greater with each passing day. I remember a time when the men's running clothes section was larger than the women's. If you have been to a running store in the last few years, you know that's not the case anymore. There are more choices for running tights than cereals in the cereal aisle at the grocery store. One more excuse to go shopping for clothes is not hurting the expansion of the running community.

We all love good food, but for the particularly refined girly girl, it is among favorite pastimes. Going out to eat at fancy restaurants is a great family activity and having a great meal is very satisfying. Although we are in an age where many men cook at home, the majority of households still have female head chefs. Being able to go out to eat is a treat for the cook, but more importantly for the runner, eating out will not pack on the pounds. Restaurant food is usually higher in calories than our home food, so the extra exercise makes those calories less noticeable.

I am convinced that God doesn't care what we look like, but He does want us to be healthy. I don't think there is anything wrong with spending time improving the way we look on the surface, but I think we have to spend time considering how we look like on the inside. Having a heart for others, taking time for prayer and Bible study and, yes, taking care of our physical bodies are important things we do to take care of what's on the inside!

- *Running may be the only time you see some ladies with little makeup and their hair not perfect!*

- *The social and fashion aspects of running have drawn more women to the sport than ever before.*

- *Taking care of our bodies is something that God tells us in important.*

running with mom

"THERE ARE NO GOOD-BYES, WHERE EVER you'll be, you'll be in my heart." - Ghandi. Life is full of stages and transitions that occur more rapidly than we sometimes realize. Some of these life phases are, for the most part, uniform for most of us in our society. Between the ages of one and two years, the ability to walk occurs. The ability to communicate with language begins to explode between the ages of two and three. Between the fifth and sixth year formal schooling begins. The period of puberty as it extends into adulthood spans the ages of ten to seventeen. There are also those stages that most go through that are not necessarily tied as much to common ages including college education, marriage and parenthood. Personal and career milestones can also transition us into different stages of life. Traumatic events such as experiencing the death of a friend or a loved one are also often common triggers for propelling individuals into new phases of life. Many phases of life, good or bad, can be at times a challenge to manage. Finding a positive way to cope with these changes can often ease the burden of the transition.

It was Mother's Day weekend when I traveled from Michigan to Iowa City for unexpected reasons. Ironically enough, it would be the first time that I had spent this special day with Mom in more than two decades. She had recently had a liver transplant and although the surgery went well and the initial outlook was positive, things had taken a turn for the worse. Although I wasn't aware of the scope of what I was about to face, I sensed that things were serious as I anticipated what was to come during the five-hour drive. When I arrived at the hospital and found my way to the ICU, the look on my dad's face and the tone in his voice told the story of what was to come.

As he and the doctor's spoke to my brother and me about my mom's fragile state and the dire odds of her recovery to live a normal healthy life, the decision was made to take Mom off of life support. My father would travel back home that afternoon to take care of some things. Upon his return back to Iowa City the next day, we would pull her from life support. The team of doctors anticipated that she would survive only a few hours after the breathing tube was taken away.

Our family would arrive a few hours later to spend the weekend with my brother and me. As children, my brother and I had seen our extended family regularly, but because of where we had settled down as adults, the distance made it difficult to keep in touch. We had only seen our uncle and two aunts a few times in the last two decades. Although Mother's Day would bring us both to a new stage in our lives, with a difficult transition, it was nice to spend the time reminiscing about childhood memories with relatives.

With the long drive and the emotional highs and lows of the day, I was exhausted by the time I arrived at the hotel room that night. After a good night's sleep, I awoke with the sunrise for a run. Although the time of conversation and group support the previous day had helped tremendously, the hour run provided some much needed isolation for me to reflect on the past and think about how my life would be different following my mother's passing. The rhythm of my heartbeat, the sound of each footfall and the sensation of sweat between my skin and clothes seemed to awaken my senses. The time of conversation with relatives just a few hours ago had offered its own therapy, but my running ritual was offering me my own private therapy session.

Like all forms of exercise, running can provide a host of physical benefits, but running can also provide a variety of mental stimulants, depending on your frame of mind. It can arouse the mind with the sights, smells, sounds and stimulus of the surrounding environment, but it can also allow the opposite to occur. An individual can tune out the external environment and tune in to one's internal stimulus while running. As I ran the streets of Iowa City on this Mother's Day, the morning skies were sunny and temperatures were mild, providing the perfect backdrop for me to explore an unfamiliar setting on the campus of the University of Iowa, but this day would not be a day of exploring a new setting for me. This run would help me to tune out the external environment and focus in on saying goodbye to my mom as I thought about this new stage in my life without her. Although I hated the thought of losing my mom on Mother's Day, I realized that her last day on earth being Mother's Day was the perfect tribute for such a dedicated and passionate mom.

Over the next few days, plans were made for a memorial service. Ironically enough, this service was scheduled for Father's Day. With a month to wait there was more than enough time to prepare, but also there was what seemed like an over abundance of time to cope with things as I anticipated my mom's funeral. Again, my running routine helped me through this time. Some of these runs helped to distract me from what was on my mind, while others tuned me in to my own emotions from positive memories to the sadness of losing a loved one. I looked forward to the weekend of the Memorial Service and the positive benefit of a family gathering as I would be reunited with relatives I had not seen in over two decades. At times, I dreaded the weekend, as well. Running seemed to help me sort through these mixed feelings not necessarily acting as a magic cure but instead providing some moments of respite.

I arrived at home five days before the memorial service. This time provided everything that I had expected as I reconnected with relatives filtering in over the next few days. My dad's intentions were to make this a time of celebration of my mom's life. His wish came true. Over the course of the long weekend, there were some tears that were shed, but for the most part, it was a time of smiles, laughter and celebration. The night before the memorial service a large crowd of family and friends gathered at the house. The only thing that could have made it any more perfect would have been if my mom were there enjoying it with us.

Similar to the experience in Iowa City a few weeks earlier, I awoke with the sunrise for a run after a day of reuniting with family. The support and conversation with family and friends the past few days had been amazing, but I had decided that some alone time the morning of the memorial service was something that I needed, as well. A two and a half hour run provided this for me. I wasn't alone, however. As I ran by the cemetery where my mom's ashes would be buried my mom ran with me. As I ran by the farmhouse where she and my dad had lived before retirement and the ground that they had farmed, Mom ran with me. As I ran by the signs that my mom and dad had made for local businesses during their years as owners of a sign shop, Mom ran with me. For two and half hours Mom ran with me.

Although I am doing well with my mom's passing, I am sure that there will be moments of sadness. I am sure the first holiday season will bring moments of grief for me. What will be most difficult is not being able to call her on the phone to tell her of the accomplishments and milestones of my own kids. She always loved hearing about her grandchildren, and I enjoyed sharing these moments with her, as well. Although I may have told Mom good-bye on Mother's Day, I know that it is not good-bye forever. If there are days when I want to tell her about something that I know she would want to hear about, or moments when I just want to spend some time with her alone, I can just go for a run with her. KEEP RUNNING!! Until next time, this has been just another runner's perspective.

Gale Fischer – *Battlecreek, MI*

Ecclesiastes 3:1-14

1 To everything there is a season,
A time for every purpose under heaven:
2 A time to be born,
And a time to die;
A time to plant,
And a time to pluck what is planted;
3 A time to kill,
And a time to heal;
A time to break down,
And a time to build up;
4 A time to weep,
And a time to laugh;
A time to mourn,
And a time to dance;
5 A time to cast away stones,
And a time to gather stones;
A time to embrace,
And a time to refrain from embracing;
6 A time to gain,
And a time to lose;
A time to keep,
And a time to throw away;
7 A time to tear,
And a time to sew;
A time to keep silence,
And a time to speak;
8 A time to love,
And a time to hate;
A time of war,
And a time of peace.

9 What profit has the worker from that in which he labors? 10 I have seen the God-given task with which the sons of men are to be occupied. 11 He has made everything beautiful in its time. Also He has put eternity in their hearts, except that no one can find out the work that God does from beginning to end.
12 I know that nothing is better for them than to rejoice, and to do good in their lives, 13 and also that every man should eat and drink and enjoy the good of all his labor—it is the gift of God.
14 I know that whatever God does,
It shall be forever.
Nothing can be added to it,
And nothing taken from it.
God does it, that men should fear before Him.

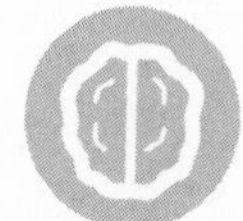

scripture memorization

Write out the scripture(s) in the space below and recite them ten times.

something to ponder

HOW OFTEN do you talk with God and loved ones without speaking a word?

DOES RUNNING help you to connect with God and help you find peace during a loss?

HOW HAS running provided emotional or spiritual therapy for you?

HAVE YOU ever set a big goal and then achieved it? Was there someone who helped you? How did they help?

DESCRIBE A time when you faced an incredible challenge and you overcame by the power of discipline, training, making a plan and keeping your eyes fixed on Jesus?

running observations

by dean

Taking Care of Your Skin

WE ALL KNOW THAT RUNNING IS good for your heart, lungs and mental health. But there are other reasons running is good for you. Studies show that regular exercise is a key to healthy skin.

So, how in the world does running help your skin? Good blood flow is important for all cells in your body to remain at their healthiest levels, including skin cells. Blood carries all the nutrients and oxygen to the working cells throughout the body to keep them as healthy as they can be. In addition, good blood flow also helps carry away waste products, like free radicals, from working cells, allowing them to work more efficiently. It's like cleaning your skin from the inside!

Running has also been known to ease stress. There are skin conditions that are exacerbated by stress, like acne and eczema. Spending time in any activity that reduces stress can improve those conditions.

Of course, there can be risks to your skin while running too. Since you spend time outside while running, sun exposure is a concern. Fortunately, protecting your skin from the sun is easy. If you do not protect your skin from the sun, you will lose all of the benefits that exercise provides for your skin. Sunburns increase your risk of skin cancer and will cause rapid aging of the skin. The best advice is to avoid running between the hours of 10 a.m. and 4 p.m. when the sun's damaging rays are at their most dangerous. If you have to run during peak sun time, wear sunscreen. Choose a sunscreen that is PH balanced so that it doesn't sting if it runs into your eyes. Also, if you have oily skin or acne, there are gel based or oil-free products available today. Last, but not least, covering your skin with clothing offers even more protection. Don't forget about your head. Wearing a hat will protect both your face and your scalp.

Another skin problem that can be brought on while running is chafing, particularly around the inside of your upper thighs, under the arms, and anywhere else your clothing rubs your skin. Although this is not a problem for everyone, it is a serious issue for some runners. If you are one of the unlucky ones who struggle with this issue, there are many products available today to help. You can find them in many places, but a running specialty store will have products made specifically for runners. The key is to find one that you like.

There are skin conditions that can be exacerbated by sweating and physical activity, but that is no excuse not to exercise. The benefits of running far outweigh the negative effects of a temporary problem. Take the time to find products that help you to be as comfortable as you can be during your runs, and you won't be sorry!

There is nothing wrong with being concerned about what your skin looks like, but it is more important to be concerned about the health of your skin. The two are not always the same. It is much like being a Christian. Just saying you're saved doesn't make it so. The Bible tells us this: Therefore, if anyone is in Christ, he is a new creation; old things have passed away; behold, all things have become new (2 Corinthians 5:17). That means you are different after you have been saved. You can look clean and say all the right things on the outside, but unless you have a healthy relationship with Jesus Christ, it's all just window dressing. How is your relationship with Him?

- *Running makes the cells of your body healthier, including your skin cells!*
- *Although there are skin conditions that are exacerbated by exercise, the benefits of running far outweigh*

the drawbacks.

- *Steady Bible study, along with a personal relationship with Jesus Christ, will make you healthy on the inside, and it will show on the outside!*

sticky notes

God and the gatorade

"AND THE GOD OF ALL GRACE, who called you to his eternal glory in Christ, after you have suffered a little while, will himself restore you and make you strong, firm and steadfast. To him be the power forever and ever. Amen." (1 Peter 5:10-11 NIV)

This was the verse God gave me for my son as he headed off to San Diego, California for a beach vacation unlike any other. Little did I know it would be my verse, too? Ben was beginning the first phase of BUD/S, part one of Navy SEAL training. Less than 20% of SEAL wannabes will graduate with their class. Phase One is the first weed-out phase. Knowing he would be pushed to limits yet unknown to him, I committed to run the Dallas Marathon in solidarity. This marked marathon number five for me, and was not my first rodeo. I knew the long miles would give me time for prayer. James 5:16 (NIV) says, "The prayer of a righteous man is powerful and effective." I figured a mom's prayer for her son was right up there with those of righteous men, so I asked God to show me how to pray.

The first training weekend, I ran a half marathon. It was nothing unusual, but the next morning found me dragging myself into church. I was so tired. What was the deal? Immediately, God spoke, "Fatigue. Pray that Ben will push through his fatigue." Wow. That was fast. Be careful what you pray for. Over the three months of training, God gave me snapshots of things Ben would deal with, such as IT Band issues and GI issues. The snapshots usually came during my long runs. One snapshot, in particular, really took me back. God blessed me with this one on a sixteen-mile run, and it hit me around mile ten. I had an overwhelming desire to stop or quit. I stopped and started for six more miles, and the truth of Ben's situation hit me. It's one thing when you have to finish. Like an out-and-back run and you just completed the out and your phone died. At least you can chill and walk a little, maybe eat something. It's far different when you have the choice to stop at any moment—and you're cold, wet, and covered in sand with instructors screaming in your ears. BUD/S trainees can DOR, drop on request, at any time. Enlisted men may try again in two years. Officers get one shot. I would later hear stories of men quitting on the next-to-the-last exercise or evolution. This one put me on my knees in prayer for days. Our training continued. Ben survived "Hell Week." Race day for me followed close behind.

The race could go one of two ways: PR, personal record, or RD, rough day. I reminded myself that this one was for Ben, and I tried not to think of a PR. Good thing, because God had RD in mind. Race day dawned warm and humid for December. I was sweating buckets by mile 2. Nausea set in at mile 10. Just looking at the food I packed made me sick adding GI issues. Lovely. Needing calories badly, I sought out the Gatorade at the next water station, which I downed. I ran as far as it took me, and struggled to the next water stop. Ten miles later, I crossed the finish line with my worst time ever. Frustrated and in tears, I refueled and headed back to Fort Worth.

After several days of pouting, God reminded me of another prayer, one I had lifted up for myself. "God, help me to learn to draw strength from You and not my flesh." I remembered. He told me He had just given me an object lesson in answer. How do you draw strength from God? One cup of Gatorade at a time. Oh. How cool is that? I stopped pouting. The author of Hebrews says this:

"Endure hardship as discipline; God is treating you as sons..... God disciplines us for our good that we may share in his holiness. No discipline seems pleasant at the time, but painful. Later on, however, it produces a harvest of righteousness and peace by those who have been trained by it." (Hebrews 12:7,10-11)

Those months marked times of training and discipline for Ben and me, but the harvest was coming. God was faithful to bring it, and for me, it was an unforgettable lesson of God and Gatorade. I love running. I love how running clears my head. I love how God speaks when I run. And I love how incredibly detailed and personal He is when He does speak. So pray and pray big. Go to Him often. Allow Him to be your trainer and your Gatorade. And when you need more, know that the refills are free. (Ben graduated with Class 298, which began with 167 men. Nineteen of those 167 graduated and received their Tridents.)

Gaye Veitenheimer – Fort Worth, TX

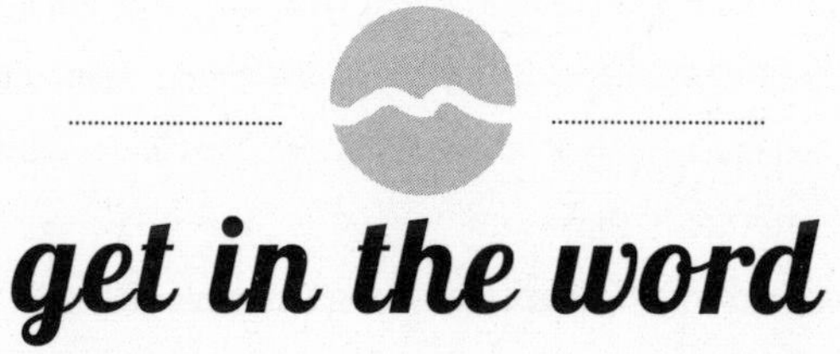

get in the word

1 Peter 5:10-11
But may the God of all grace, who called us to His eternal glory by Christ Jesus, after you have suffered a while, perfect, establish, strengthen, and settle you. To Him be the glory and the dominion forever and ever. Amen.

James 5:16
Confess your trespasses to one another, and pray for one another, that you may be healed. The effective, fervent prayer of a righteous man avails much.

Hebrews 12:7, 10-11
If you endure chastening, God deals with you, as with sons; for what son is there whom a father does not chasten?
For they indeed for a few days chastened us as seemed best to them,

but He for our profit, that we may be partakers of His holiness. Now no chastening seems to be joyful for the present, but painful; nevertheless, afterward it yields the peaceable fruit of righteousness to those who have been trained by it.

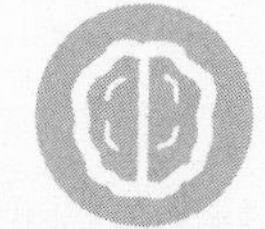

scripture memorization

Write out the scripture(s) in the space below and recite them ten times.

something to ponder

DO YOU believe God has a purpose in the hard times, or do you think He is out to get you?

DO YOU believe God will speak to you?

IS YOUR relationship with God a cup-by-cup thing or are you dying of thirst?

running observations by dean

Excessive Celebration

I REMEMBER, BACK IN 1988, WHEN running back Ickey Woods scored a touchdown in an NFL game, he would perform a short dance, which came to be known as the "Ickey Shuffle." I thought it was fun to watch, and we would view Cincinnati Bengals games just to see him score, which he did 18 times in his rookie season. There were some before him and many after him who became famous for their antics after they scored. Eventually, the NFL saw this as a distraction from the game and the practice now results in a penalty and even an individual fine for the offending player. Still, players are allowed to show some excitement so long as it is not a choreographed routine or considered taunting an opposing player. There is some gray area left open to interpretation by the officials.

Is there such a thing as excessive celebration in running? Sure, there is, but more often we shortchange our celebration.

There is a fine line between bragging and sharing. I love to see a Facebook post about a friend's race result, but how it's presented means everything. If it comes across as "Hey, look how great I am!" it is excessive celebration, sort of like taunting in football. However, if it comes across as "I'd like you to share in my accomplishment!" I would call it a fair play. Like football, there is a gray area, left up to those who read the post as the officials. We don't know how our friends and acquaintances are going to react when we talk about our accomplishments so we cheat on the side of saying less.

Humbleness is a great trait, but we should celebrate milestones in our lives. If you think about it, sharing those accomplishments will often inspire or even challenge others. Can you remember a time when someone shared their success with you and it made you want to go out and do the same thing? Maybe your first 5K came after you had heard about someone else. You thought, "If she can do it, so can I." You don't want to deprive someone else of the motivation they need to get up and going, do you? You may not want to stand up on a table in the middle of a crowded room and declare that you crushed Sally by a full minute this weekend, but making sure your friends know that you ran a PR this past weekend is absolutely necessary! Timing, of course, is important. You may want to wait until it comes up naturally in conversation instead of interrupting someone in the middle of their movie review from Saturday night. That might be considered excessive celebration!

Is there such a thing as excessive celebration when it comes to sharing Christ with others? At first glance, it seems that the answer might be no, but take a second look. The Bible tells us that we are to minister to others' needs as a priority. When someone is down and in a dark place in life, the last thing they want to hear is about how happy and filled with the Spirit someone else is. In John 15:13 Jesus said, "Greater love has no one than this: to lay down one's life for one's friends." He is not telling us that we have to die for others, but that we should put the needs of others ahead of our own. Once we have done that, there is almost always a time for sharing in your celebrations with others!

- *There is a fine line between bragging and sharing, and there is a lot of gray area that is open to interpretation by the listener.*

- *Never forget that your accomplishments may be the spark that gets someone else going!*

- *Living by Jesus' words in John 15:13 as a priority in our lives will give us more friends to celebrate all of life's high points with in the future!*

sticky notes

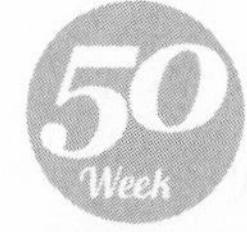

keep my eyes on Jesus

WHEN I STARTED THE RUN FOR God class at my church, I was a novice runner, to say the least. I ran a local 5K once a year and thought I was awesome. I also thought I was pretty sure about how life was supposed to be. Yes, I knew I was saved, but my walk with God wasn't what it should be. As the class progressed, and we started running for five minute intervals, I soon found myself struggling to keep up. Each time I would complain, my class leader would remind me to pray and let God help me get through it and to have faith. I took her words and half-heartedly put them to use. I pressed on and somehow made it each time, and each time, I barely had a breath left to finish, but I finished. I finished. I was so proud of ME for making it to almost 10 minutes of nonstop running.

When it came time for the day of 20 minutes of running, suddenly I had the urge to tackle this myself. I decided to have a night run in the neighborhood. It was summer and it was still hot after nine o'clock at night, but I enjoyed evening running. It was peaceful and I could talk to God and just enjoy the sounds of summer. I was about two or three minutes into the run when I started having trouble. My legs started to hurt and I felt lousy. Immediately, I knew I wouldn't be making the 20 minute run, and I wasn't sure if I'd even make a 10 minute jog, so I kept on despite the pain and discomfort and continued to feel worse. Suddenly, I started to pray.

I felt burdened with myself and how I had been behaving. It was like God was showing me how prideful I'd been, how I'd been trying to do it all on my own, and that it wasn't going to end the way I wanted it to if I kept on. He was showing me that I needed Him, not only in running, but also in life. In that moment, my eyes were opened, and I could see and hear clearly. The struggle I was having in my running wasn't just because I was out of shape or not ready to progress to 20 minutes, it was because I'd taken the focus off Jesus and put it on myself. I began to weep and ask forgiveness of my sin and begged Jesus to help me in life and in running. I asked HIM to carry me the rest of the way and help me do it with His help - and, that is just what He did.

As I continued to run, an overwhelming feeling of peace came upon me, and my strength was renewed. The aching of my legs disappeared and my body felt at ease. At one point, I wasn't even sure if my feet were touching the ground because my run became so amazing. I stayed in constant prayer and thanksgiving for the rest of the 20 minutes and began to pace myself and chant under my breath "keep my eyes on Jesus...keep my eyes on Jesus." I kept that rhythm for the rest of the run. It was an awesome, unbelievable experience that night. Even though not all my runs are like this, I find that when I do keep my eyes on Jesus and stay in prayer with Him, I am able to complete my runs. Just this past weekend, I completed my first 5K since graduating the 5k class, and He carried me through, yet again, and helped me cross the finish line with a time nine minutes better than my personal record. It's all about Him...it's all about Jesus.

Kim Langley – *Searcy, AR*

get in the word

Philippians 4:13

I can do all things through Christ who strengthens me.

Hebrews 12:1

Therefore we also, since we are surrounded by so great a cloud of witnesses, let us lay aside every weight, and the sin which so easily ensnares us, and let us run with endurance the race that is set before us,

Colossians 3:2

Set your mind on things above, not on things on the earth.

scripture memorization

Write out the scripture(s) in the space below and recite them ten times.

something to ponder

WHY DOES my faith sometimes waiver?

WHAT IS it that keeps me from focusing on God?

WHY DO I sometimes think I can do it all without His help?

running observations by dean

Ever Thought About a Triathlon?

DOES THE THOUGHT OF A TRIATHLON intrigue you or does it overwhelm you? Or, does it intrigue you and then overwhelm you? Most runners have definite thoughts about a triathlon and they are either eager to try one or have no interest in them. My first thought, before completing one, was the dread of the water. I'm a runner and not a swimmer. Since swimming is so much different than running, there are few people who are good at both. But, I had a bucket list item to cross off the list, so I took the plunge, pun intended. I learned some things.

First, I learned that triathlons are for everyone. Many years ago, it was thought that running a marathon was only for seriously dedicated lifetime runners. Today, we know that almost anyone can conquer the marathon with enough motivation and hard work. It may not be easy, but more and more average Joes complete marathons every year. The thoughts about completing over twenty-six miles had to evolve over time. I think we are in the middle stages of triathlon evolution now. There are not as many triathlons as marathons, but the number is increasing, and there are likely more out there than you think. If you have thought that these races are only for fast people, or professionals, you may want to re-evaluate your notion of what a triathlon looks like. If you have never been to a triathlon, find one close by to go watch and you'll be amazed how many people in the race look like you do!

Second, I learned that you don't have to give up your life to train for a triathlon. Just because you're participating in three different disciplines does not mean you have to do three times the training. You can expect to spend more time training simply because swimming and cycling are not as efficient as running. What I mean by that is that you can lace up your running shoes and start running from your front door. Depending upon where you live, you may or may not be able to do that on a bicycle, but either way, cycling takes more time than running. A six mile run that may take me forty-five minutes is roughly equal to a twenty mile bike ride that will take an hour. Swimming may not take any longer than running, but most people have to travel somewhere to do it. But, if you're creative in scheduling, you can fit in all of it, and it doesn't have to feel much more difficult than trying to run every day.

Another thing you may not know about triathlons is that they vary in distances just like running events. You don't have to begin by thinking about a race that takes many hours. There are a number of "super sprint" triathlons that can be completed in less than an hour and a half. A super sprint distance triathlon is defined as being shorter than a sprint triathlon. If the swim bothers you, many of these short triathlons take place in the safety of a pool. Many of these races cater to beginners and they are a great way to get your feet wet, pun intended again! The standard distances for longer triathlons are: Sprint – 750 meter swim, 20 kilometer bike, 5K run; Olympic – 1500 meter swim, 40 kilometer bike, 10K run; Half Ironman – 1.2 mile swim, 56 mile bike, half marathon run; Ironman – 2.4 mile swim, 112 mile bike, marathon run. But there are many other distances, short and long, including "ultra-triathlons" which are even longer than an Ironman distance. Those are reserved for crazy people!

When George Mallory was asked why he wanted to climb Mount Everest, he famously replied, "Because it's there." Perhaps you don't need any other reason than this to try your first triathlon. They are there, waiting for you!

Why should you worship the one true God? Because He's there! What separates God from others is that our God is alive. He's there and He sent his son to die for our sins. Romans 5:8 says, “But God demonstrates His own love toward us, in that while we were still sinners, Christ died for us.” He wants and deserves our worship. Unlike a triathlon or a mountain that you must travel to, God will meet you wherever you are. He's right there where you are, right now! No swimming required.

- *Triathlons are for everyone.*
- *There are triathlons that cater to newbies.*
- *Worship God because of what He did for you because He's there!*

sticky notes

51
Week

the finish line

WELL, AFTER 12 WEEKS OF TRAINING, tonight is our Hopewell Hustle 5K. I am excited and ready for it! God has given us perfect weather to run. As I reflect over these past 12 weeks, I can't help but remember how I thought running for 60 seconds was so hard. I could barely catch my breath and, after many Ibuprofen and ice packs to various parts of my body, I am now prepared to run 3.1 miles.

It hasn't been easy, but it has been worth it. I am thankful for so many things that I have experienced during these 12 weeks: the awesome leadership of the Run for God program at Hopewell, old friendships that have become stronger, the formation of new friendships, the encouragement from each and every member of the group, my Brooks running shoes, Gatorade, the weight loss I have achieved (down 19.5 lbs.), and more importantly, the love and support from my wonderful husband and daughter as we went through this journey together. Most importantly, none of this would have been possible if it were not for Jesus.

My go-to verse throughout this process has been Philippians 4:13, NKJV: "I can do ALL things through Christ who strengthens me." Just last week, my mother-in-law passed away. As we watched her take her final breath, I knew without a doubt that she had entered Heaven. She ran her final race, and she crossed the best finish line ever. Tonight, I will run my race to the best of my ability and give God all the glory for it.

Jennifer Camden – *Monroe, NC*

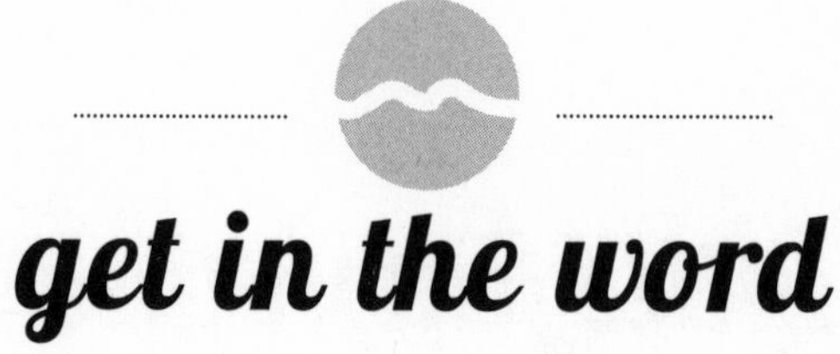

get in the word

Philippians 4:13

I can do all things through Christ who strengthens me.

Hebrews 12:1

Therefore we also, since we are surrounded by so great a cloud of witnesses, let us lay aside every weight, and the sin, which so easily ensnares us, and let us run with endurance the race that is set before us.

Isaiah 40:31

But those who wait on the Lord shall renew their strength; they shall mount up with wings like eagles, they shall run and not be weary, they shall walk and not faint.

scripture memorization

Write out the scripture(s) in the space below and recite them ten times.

something to ponder

WHERE WILL you be when you cross your finish line?

____

____

____

____

____

HOW WILL you run your race?

____

____

____

____

____

HAVE YOU put your trust in the Lord?

____

____

____

running observations by dean

Running on Vacation

THERE ARE MANY WAYS TO SPEND your free time away from work and the grind of daily life. Some vacationers enjoy going to the beach and just relaxing for hours, even days, at a time. My wife and I love to drive around the country and have taken vacations where we have driven over 3,500 miles in nine days, packing our days with anything and everything we come across on our journey. Whether you enjoy the relaxation and calm of a mountain retreat or like to experience new adventures while on vacation, running can be a part of any vacation.

Some runners like to take time off from running and it's a good idea to do that occasionally, but I'm not sure vacation time is the best time to do it. After all, many of us run because it's something we love to do, so why would we stop when we are supposed to be doing things we love to do? I'm going to try to make the case for running on vacation.

First, and maybe most importantly, running is one of the best ways to see a city or town. I like to get up early, lace up my shoes and explore the area around our hotel. The route I choose is dependent upon whether we are at a new destination or someplace we have been before. When we have chosen a new stop, I run around the main streets of the town looking for places to eat and things to do that we may not have thought about on our way. It's rare that I am disappointed by what I find. If we are in a familiar city, I like to explore the nooks and crannies of the city. I am often disappointed on these runs, not because of what I find, but because I rarely take a camera with me and there is nearly always something to photograph!

Secondly, there's something so peaceful about running around a city before it wakes up. When Debbie and I went to Las Vegas, our plane arrived after 11:00 p.m. We checked into the hotel and decided to walk down the streets at midnight, because we didn't know any better. If you have been to Las Vegas, you may know that the late night atmosphere is less than family friendly. As we walked down the street, looking for something to eat, we discussed what a mistake we made in going to Sin City. We went back to our hotel and thought we would spend more time at the Grand Canyon than we had planned, but a funny thing happened when I went for a run in the morning. I got up early despite our late arrival and it hit me as soon as I went out the door, the city was so still. Not only that, but all of the trash that had been strewn all over the sidewalks was cleaned up and the city looked like a completely different place. As it turned out, it was a different place when the sun was out. After scouting the city and getting the lay of the land, it began to wake. The difference was that the late night partiers were all replaced by families! We went to bed early that night. If I were not a runner, I would have missed part of the city's transformation.

Third, it's a great excuse to take it easy and do what you want. If you want to run easy, do it. If you want to stop and gaze at the ocean, do it. If you want to walk for a little while, do it. All the running rules are out the window and your goal is to make it as fun as you can. I look forward to vacation runs, because they're fun. I only wear a watch on these runs to know how long I have been running. I turn the GPS off. I don't want to be enticed to run farther or harder than I want. After all, it's my vacation.

Finally, if you have never taken a running vacation, I highly recommend it! Choose a race based on the destination, sign up and take a Runcation! There are races in every destination city, and they are often at non-peak times, so accommodations are less expensive. Make sure you leave plenty of time for vacation exploration. Look at it this way; if you have a bad race, you still have vacation time!

It's refreshing to experience running in a new and different way and vacation running is a great way to do just that. It's also exciting to experience God in new and different ways. Has your quiet time with God become stale at times? Falling into a habit of going through the motions is human nature. Just like running on vacation provides a change of scenery and excuses to do it differently, Bible study can be changed to make it fresh. For example, if you typically read a few chapters a day, try finding one verse and focus on it for days. If you follow a plan, try going your own direction by finding something in your study Bible that piques your interest. While on vacation, go to a different church. A vacation rejuvenates us because it is different from the daily grind. Changing your Bible study and prayer habits from time to time will make things look fresh again!

- *Running while on vacation provides a different look at the city or town you are visiting.*

- *Runcations will inject excitement into your running.*

- *When things get too repetitive in your daily quiet time, change things up to experience Him in a new and different way.*

sticky notes

stay a little longer

"YOU'D COME IN THIRD IN A race with a pregnant woman." Growing up, my dad told me that more times than I care to remember. Once was more than enough. Despite my God-given athletic ability, (I could throw a fastball that made my catcher have to wear weight-lifting gloves, so her hands would bruise 'just' purple instead of black. I had a sweet spot on my bat that sent balls deep into the outfield). I wasn't a fast runner, and he let me know it.

Twenty years later, I still hear those words reverberating in my ears. My face still burns hot and tears sting my eyes with shame. In fact, those words kept me sitting on the sidelines for years. I'd laugh, "If you see me running, you better run, too, because something's chasing me," but, secretly and longingly, I would watch runners out of the corner of my eye. I had romantic notions of running through the streets of my small town, enjoying the beauty and crispness of fall. How I longed to run. There seemed to be such freedom in running, but fear kept me on the sidelines, frozen. Replaying those words over and over. I didn't want to embarrass myself, and then, I submitted.

Submission is a funny thing. I wrestle God with something, in this case, running, and I know I will give in eventually and when I do, submission is so freeing, and I wonder why I was holding on for so long to whatever He wanted me to let go of. So, I let go of the sidelines, and when I did, I found the freedom I'd been looking for. At first, I dreaded how I'd look coming in to the church after a group Run for God run, sweat dripping off my late-teen sized body. I begged God, "Anything but this." Having my trainer/teacher/cheerleader rub my legs, one at a time, while I lay on the floor, one leg in the air, writhing in pain of shin splints as others looked on and said, "You'll feel so much better soon!" The sweet freedom of submission was worth trading my pride.

When I first began those weeks of running a minute, I felt shame. My Jesus suffered the agony of the cross, and I was wondering how I was going to make it through forty-five more seconds of running. My face burned hot and tears stung my eyes. I would press on. As the time increased each week and my endurance was put to the test, I would say over and over, "I can do all things through Christ who gives me strength," and as the weeks wore on, and I still used that verse, especially to get me going or in the final minutes as I tried to reach my goal, I started to notice a change. Instead of asking with dread, "How much longer?", I began asking the same question with hope, starting my stopwatch, taking off, and whooping with delight when I discovered I had run longer than ever before. When I began to wonder how much farther God would carry me during my runs, I began to hear Him whisper to my soul, "You're not who others say you are. You are who I say you are." Instead of the stinging words from my earthly father, I hear my heavenly Daddy saying, "Run with Me a little longer. Talk to Me a little longer. Tell Me your worries. Praise Me. Ask Me. Share with Me. A little longer."

The amazing thing is this. When I submit to His prompting to "stay a little longer", I find that it's not just time added to my physical endurance. He's adding to my endurance in all areas of my life. Things I never dreamed I'd be able to get through or endure aren't as daunting. I am able with Him, through Him, and because of Him. When I "stay a little longer", my endurance is put to the test and I'm pushed beyond limits I'd never dreamed possible for myself; I come to the end of myself and enter the beginning of Him. He doesn't care how fast or slow I run because I'm delighting in my time with Him, and He is delighting in His time with me. I'm always so glad I "stayed a little longer".